Evidence-based Clinical Chinese Medicine

Volume 12
Post-Stroke Shoulder Complications

Evidence-based Clinical Chinese Medicine

Co Editors-in-Chief

Charlie Changli Xue
RMIT University, Australia

Chuanjian Lu
Guangdong Provincial Hospital of Chinese Medicine, China

Volume 12

Post-Stroke Shoulder Complications

Lead Authors

Claire Shuiqing Zhang
RMIT University, Australia

Shaonan Liu
Guangdong Provincial Hospital of Chinese Medicine, China

World Scientific

NEW JERSEY · LONDON · SINGAPORE · BEIJING · SHANGHAI · HONG KONG · TAIPEI · CHENNAI · TOKYO

Published by

World Scientific Publishing Co. Pte. Ltd.

5 Toh Tuck Link, Singapore 596224

USA office: 27 Warren Street, Suite 401-402, Hackensack, NJ 07601

UK office: 57 Shelton Street, Covent Garden, London WC2H 9HE

Library of Congress Cataloging-in-Publication Data
Names: Xue, Charlie Changli, author. | Lu, Chuan-jian, 1964–   author.
Title: Evidence-based clinical Chinese medicine / Charlie Changli Xue, Chuanjian Lu.
Description: New Jersey : World Scientific, 2016. | Includes bibliographical references and index.
Identifiers: LCCN 2015030389| ISBN 9789814723084 (v. 1 : hardcover : alk. paper) |
    ISBN 9789814723091 (v. 1 : paperback : alk. paper) |
    ISBN 9789814723121 (v. 2 : hardcover : alk. paper) |
    ISBN 9789814723138 (v. 2 : paperback : alk. paper) |
    ISBN 9789814759045 (v. 3 : hardcover : alk. paper) |
    ISBN 9789814759052 (v. 3 : paperback : alk. paper)
Subjects: | MESH: Medicine, Chinese Traditional--methods. | Clinical Medicine--methods. |
    Evidence-Based Medicine--methods. | Psoriasis. | Pulmonary Disease, Chronic Obstructive.
Classification: LCC RC81 | NLM WB 55.C4 | DDC 616--dc23
LC record available at http://lccn.loc.gov/2015030389

Volume 12: Post-Stroke Shoulder Complications
ISBN 978-981-120-759-4

British Library Cataloguing-in-Publication Data
A catalogue record for this book is available from the British Library.

Copyright © 2020 by World Scientific Publishing Co. Pte. Ltd.

For any available supplementary material, please visit
https://www.worldscientific.com/worldscibooks/10.1142/11481#t=suppl

Disclaimer

The information in this book is based on systematic analyses of the best available evidence for Chinese medicine interventions, both historical and contemporary. Every effort has been made to ensure accuracy and completeness of the data herein. This book is intended for clinicians, researchers and educators. The practice of evidence-based medicine consists of consideration of the best available evidence, practitioners' clinical experience and judgment, and patients' preference. Not all interventions are acceptable in all countries. It is important to note that some of the substances mentioned in this book may no longer be in use, may be toxic, or may be prohibited or restricted under the provisions of the Convention on International Trade in Endangered Species of Wild Fauna and Flora (CITES). Practitioners, researchers and educators are advised to comply with the relevant regulations in their country and with the restrictions on the trade in species included in CITES appendices I, II and III. This book is not intended as a guide for self-medication. Patients should seek professional advice from qualified Chinese medicine practitioners.

Foreword

Since the late 20th century, Chinese medicine, including acupuncture and herbal medicine, has been increasingly used throughout the world. The parallel development and spread of evidence-based medicine has provided challenges and opportunities for Chinese medicine. The opportunities have been evidence-based medicine's emphasis on the effective use of the best available clinical evidence, incorporating the clinicians' clinical experience, subject to patients' preference. Such practices have a patient focus which reflects the historical nature of Chinese medicine practice. However, the challenges are also significant due to the fact that, despite the long-term development and very rich literature accumulated over 2,000 years, there is an overall lack of high-level clinical evidence for many of the interventions used in Chinese medicine.

To address this knowledge gap, we need to generate clinical evidence through high-quality clinical studies and to evaluate evidence to enable effective use of such available evidence to promote evidence-based Chinese medicine practice.

Modern Chinese medicine is rooted in its classical literature and the legacies of ancient doctors, grounded in practice of expert clinicians and increasingly informed by clinical and experimental research efforts. In recognition of the unique features of Chinese medicine, for each of the conditions in this series a 'whole-evidence' approach is used to provide a synthesis of different types and levels of evidence to enable practitioners to make clinical decisions informed by the current best evidence.

There are four main components of this 'whole-evidence' approach. In the first component, we present the current approaches to the diagnosis, differentiation and treatment of each condition based on expert consensus of textbooks and clinical guidelines. This provides an overview of how the condition is currently managed. The second component provides an analysis of the condition in historical context based on systematic searches of the *Zhong Hua Yi Dian* which includes the full texts of more than 1,000 classical medical books. These analyses provide objective views on how the condition has been treated over two millennia, reveal continuities and discontinuities between traditional and modern practice, and suggest avenues for future research.

The third component is the assessment of evidence derived from modern clinical studies of Chinese medicine interventions. The methods established by the *Cochrane Collaboration* are used for conducting systematic reviews and undertaking meta-analyses of outcome data for randomised controlled trials (RCTs). In addition, the clinical relevance of meta-analysis data is enhanced by examining the herbal formulas, individual herbs and acupuncture treatments that were assessed in the RCTs, and the evidence base is broadened by the inclusion of data from controlled clinical trials and non-controlled studies. The fourth component is to determine how the herbal medicine interventions may achieve the effects indicated by the clinical trials. Thus for each of the most frequently used herbs we provide reviews of their effects in pre-clinical models and their likely mechanisms of action.

For each condition, this 'whole-evidence' approach links clinical expertise, historical precedent, clinical research data and experimental research to provide the reader with assessments of the current state of the evidence of efficacy and safety for Chinese medicine interventions using herbal medicines, acupuncture and moxibustion and other health care practices such as *taichi*.

Since these books are available in Chinese and English, they can benefit patients, practitioners and educators internationally and enable practitioners to make clinical decisions informed by the current best evidence.

These publications represent a major milestone in Chinese medicine development and make a significant contribution to the evidence-based Chinese medicine development globally.

Co-editors-in-Chief

Professor Charlie Changli Xue, RMIT University, Australia

Professor Chuanjian Lu, Guangdong Provincial Hospital of Chinese Medicine, China

Purpose of This Book

This book is intended for clinicians, researchers and educators. It can be used to inform tertiary education and clinical practice by providing systematic, multidimensional assessments of the best available evidence for using Chinese medicine to manage each common clinical condition.

How to Use This Book

Some Definitions

A glossary is included, containing terms and definitions which frequently appear in the book. It also describes the definitions of statistical tests, methodological terms, evaluation tools and interventions. For example, in this book, integrative medicine refers to the combined use of a Chinese medicine treatment with conventional medical management, and combination therapies refer to two or more Chinese medicines from different therapy groups (e.g. Chinese herbal medicine, acupuncture or other Chinese medicine therapies) administered together. Terminology used throughout the book is based on the World Health Organisation's *Standard Terminologies on Traditional Medicine in the Western Pacific Region* (2007) where possible or from the cited reference.

Data Analysis and Interpretation of Results

In order to synthesise the clinical evidence, a range of statistical analysis approaches are used. In general, the effect size for dichotomous data is reported as a risk ratio (RR) with 95% confidence interval (CI), and for continuous data, they are reported as mean difference (MD) with 95% CI. Statistically significant effects are indicated with an asterisk*. Readers should note that statistical significance does not necessarily correspond with a clinically important effect. Interpretation of results should take into consideration the clinical significance, quality of studies (expressed as high, low or unclear risk of bias in this book) and heterogeneity amongst the studies. Tests for heterogeneity are conducted using the I^2 statistic. An I^2 score greater than 50% was considered to indicate substantial heterogeneity.

Use of Evidence in Practice

The Grading of Recommendations Assessment, Development and Evaluation (GRADE) approach was used to summarise the quality of evidence and results of the strength of evidence for critical and important comparisons and outcomes. Due to the diverse nature of Chinese medicine practice, treatment recommendations are not included with the summary of findings tables. Therefore readers will need to interpret the evidence with reference to the local practice environment.

Limitations

Readers should note some of the methodological limitations on classical literature and clinical evidence.

- Search terms used to search the *Zhong Hua Yi Dian* database may not include all terms that have been used for the condition, which may alter the findings;
- Chinese language has changed over time. Citations have been interpreted for analysis, and such interpretations may be subject to disagreement;
- Chinese medicine theory has evolved over time. As such, concepts described in classical Chinese medical literature may no longer be found in contemporary works.

- Symptoms described in citations may be common to many conditions, and a judgment was required to determine the likelihood of the citation being related to the condition. This may have introduced some bias due to the subjective nature of the judgment.
- The vast majority of the clinical evidence for Chinese medicine treatments has come from China. The applicability of the findings to other populations and other countries requires further assessment.
- Many studies included participants with varying disease severity. Where possible, subgroup analyses were undertaken to examine the effects in different subpopulations. As this was not always possible, the findings may be limited to the population included, and not to subpopulations.
- The potential risk of bias found in many included studies suggested methodological limitations. The findings for GRADE assessments based on studies of very low to moderate quality evidence should be interpreted accordingly.
- Nine major English and Chinese language databases were searched to identify clinical studies, in addition to clinical trial registers. Other studies may exist which were not identified through searches, and which may alter the findings.
- The calculation of frequency of herbal formula use was based on formula names only. It is possible that studies evaluated herbal treatments with the same or similar herb ingredients, but which were given different formula names. Due to the complexity of herbal formulas, it was considered not appropriate to make a judgment as to the similarity of formulas for analysis. As such, the frequency of formulas reported in Chapter 5 may be underestimated.
- The most frequently utilised herbs which may have contributed to the treatment effect have been described in Chapter 5. These herbs may provide leads for further exploration. Calculation of the herbs with potential effect is based on frequency of formulas reported in the studies, and does not take into consideration the clinical implications and functions of every herb in a formula.

Authors and Contributors

CO-EDITORS-IN-CHIEF

Prof. Charlie Changli Xue (*RMIT University, Australia*)
Prof. Chuanjian Lu (*Guangdong Provincial Hospital of Chinese Medicine, China*)

CO-DEPUTY EDITORS-IN-CHIEF

A/Prof. Anthony Lin Zhang (*RMIT University, Australia*)
Dr. Brian H May (*RMIT University, Australia*)
Prof. Xinfeng Guo (*Guangdong Provincial Hospital of Chinese Medicine, China*)
Prof. Zehuai Wen (*Guangdong Provincial Hospital of Chinese Medicine, China*)

LEAD AUTHORS

Dr. Claire Shuiqing Zhang (*RMIT University, Australia*)
Dr. Shaonan Liu (*Guangdong Provincial Hospital of Chinese Medicine, China*)

CO-AUTHORS

RMIT University (Australia):
Dr. Shefton Parker
A/Prof. Anthony Lin Zhang
Prof. Charlie Changli Xue

Guangdong Provincial Hospital of Chinese Medicine (China):
Dr. Yiyi Cai
Dr. Ruihuan Pan

Prof. Youhua Guo
Prof. Hongxia Chen
Prof. Xinfeng Guo
Prof. Zehuai Wen
Prof. Chuanjian Lu

Members of Advisory Committee and Panel

CO-CHAIRS OF PROJECT PLANNING COMMITTEE

Prof. Peter J Coloe (*RMIT University, Australia*)
Prof. Yubo Lyu (*Guangdong Provincial Hospital of Chinese Medicine, China*)
Prof. Dacan Chen (*Guangdong Provincial Hospital of Chinese Medicine, China*)

CENTRE ADVISORY COMMITTEE (IN ALPHABETICAL ORDER)

Prof. Keji Chen (*The Chinese Academy of Sciences, China*)
Prof. Aiping Lu (*Hong Kong Baptist University, China*)
Prof. Caroline Smith (*University of Western Sydney, Australia*)
Prof. David F Story (*RMIT University, Australia*)

METHODOLOGY EXPERT ADVISORY PANEL (IN ALPHABETICAL ORDER)

Prof. Zhaoxiang Bian (*Hong Kong Baptist University, China*)
The late Prof. George Lewith (*University of Southampton, United Kingdom*)
Prof. Lixing Lao (*The University of Hong Kong, China*)
Prof. Jianping Liu (*Beijing University of Chinese Medicine, China*)
Prof. Frank Thien (*Monash University, Australia*)
Prof. Jialiang Wang (*Sichuan University, China*)

CONTENT EXPERT ADVISORY PANEL (IN ALPHABETICAL ORDER)

Prof. Jongbae Jay Park (*Department of Anesthesiology Center for Translational Pain Medicine, Duke University, USA*)

Prof. Linpeng Wang (*Beijing Hospital of Chinese Medicine, China*)

Prof. Zehuai Wen (*Guangdong Provincial Hospital of Chinese Medicine, China*)

Prof. Guoqing Zheng (*The Second Affiliation Hospital of Wenzhou Medical University, China*)

Professor Charlie Changli Xue

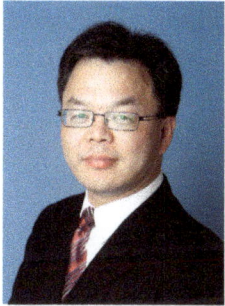

Professor Charlie Changli Xue holds a Bachelor of Medicine (majoring in Chinese Medicine) from Guangzhou University of Chinese Medicine, China (1987) and a PhD from RMIT University, Australia (2000). He has been an academic, researcher, regulator and practitioner for almost three decades. Professor Xue has made significant contributions to evidence-based educational development, clinical research, regulatory framework and policy development, and provision of high-quality clinical care to the community. Professor Xue is recognised internationally as an expert in evidence-based traditional medicine and integrative health care.

Professor Xue is the Inaugural National Chair of the Chinese Medicine Board of Australia appointed by the Australian Health Workforce Ministerial Council in 2011, and he was reappointed for a second term in 2014. Since 2007, he has been a Member of the World Health Organisation (WHO) Expert Advisory Panel for Traditional and Complementary Medicine, Geneva. Professor Xue is also Honorary Senior Principal Research Fellow at the Guangdong Provincial Academy of Chinese Medical Sciences, China.

At RMIT, Professor Xue is Executive Dean, School of Health and Biomedical Sciences. He is also Director of the WHO Collaborating Centre for Traditional Medicine.

Between 1995 and 2010, Professor Xue was Discipline Head of Chinese Medicine at RMIT University. He leads the development of five successful undergraduate and postgraduate degree programmes in Chinese Medicine at RMIT University which is now a global leader in Chinese medicine education and research.

Professor Xue's research has been supported by over AU$15 million research grants including six project grants from the Australian Government's National Health and Medical Research Council (NHMRC) and two Australian Research Council (ARC) grants. He has contributed over 200 publications and has been frequently invited as keynote speaker for numerous national and international conferences. Professor Xue has contributed to over 300 media interviews on issues related to complementary medicine education, research, regulation and practice.

Professor Chuanjian Lu

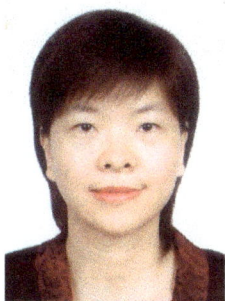

Professor Chuanjian Lu, Doctor of Medicine, is the Vice-president of Guangdong Provincial Hospital of Chinese Medicine (Guangdong Provincial Academy of Chinese Medical Sciences, Second Clinical Medical College of Guangzhou University of Chinese Medicine). She is also the Chair of the Guangdong Traditional Chinese Medicine (TCM) Standardisation Technical Committee, and the Vice-chair of the Immunity Specialty Committee of the World Federation of Chinese Medicine Societies (WFCMS).

Professor Lu has engaged in scientific research into TCM, clinical practice and teaching for some 25 years. Her research has been devoted to integrated traditional and western medicine. She has edited and published 12 monographs and 120 academic research articles as first author and corresponding author with over 30 articles being included in SCI journals. She has received widespread recognition for her achievements with awards for Excellent Teacher of South China, National Outstanding Women TCM Doctor and National Outstanding Young Doctor of TCM. She also received the Science and Technology Star of the Association of Chinese Medicine, the National Excellent Science and Technology Workers of China Award and the Five-continent Women's Scientific Awards of China Medical Women's Association.

Professor Lu has won the Award of Science and Technology Progress over ten times from Guangdong Provincial Government, China Association of Chinese Medicine and Chinese Hospital Association.

Acknowledgements

The authors and contributors would like to acknowledge the valuable contribution of research assistants and students who assisted with database searches, data extraction, data screening, data assessment, translation of documents, editing, and/or administrative tasks: Dr. Jhodie Duncan, Ms. Aiping Li, Ms. Ruzhuang Liang, Ms. Jingmin Lu, Dr. George Shengxi Zhang, Ms. Jingwen Zhu, Ms. Ke Zhu, and Mr. Jinhong Zuo.

Contents

Contents

List of Figures

List of Tables

1

Introduction to Post-stroke Shoulder Complications

OVERVIEW

Shoulder complications are common for stroke patients. This chapter reviews three main post-stroke shoulder complications (shoulder subluxation, shoulder pain and shoulder-hand syndrome) with respect to its definition, epidemiology, classification, diagnosis, clinical management and prognosis.

Introduction

Stroke was defined by the World Health Organisation (WHO) in 1989 as 'developing clinical signs of focal (or global) disturbance of cerebral function, with symptoms lasting 24 hours or longer or leading to death, with no apparent cause other than of vascular origin'.[1] Strokes can be classified into two major categories: ischaemic and haemorrhagic. Ischaemic strokes are caused by interruption of the blood supply to the brain, while haemorrhagic strokes result from the rupture of a blood vessel or an abnormal vascular structure.

According to a WHO global status report on non-communicable diseases, around 6.7 million deaths were caused by stroke in 2012; thus, it is the third most common cause of death in developed countries, exceeded only by coronary heart disease and cancer.[2] Despite the high mortality rate, it had been estimated that around 40% of stroke patients were left with moderate functional impairments and 15–30% with severe disability.[3] Worldwide, 15 million people suffer a stroke each year; one-third die and one-third are left permanently disabled.[2] With the increase of an ageing population, it is expected that the global burden of stroke will also rise, with five million permanently disabled each year, placing a huge burden on families and communities. Guidelines for Adult Stroke Rehabilitation and Recovery produced by the American Heart Association/American Stroke Association[4] reported that, between 2000 and 2010, each year stroke affects nearly 800,000 individuals in the United States, with many survivors experiencing persistent difficulty with daily tasks as a direct consequence. In Australia, stroke is one of the biggest killers and a leading cause of disability; 65% of those living with stroke also suffer a disability that impedes their ability to carry out daily living activities unassisted.[5] In 2012 there were over 420,000 people living with the effects of stroke with 30% of these people being of working age, and the total financial costs of stroke in Australia in 2012 was estimated to be $5 billion AUD.[6]

In China, with its current population of 1.4 billion, the annual stroke mortality rate is approximately 1.6 million, approximately 157 per 100,000, which has exceeded heart disease to become the leading cause of death and adult disability. In addition, China has 2.5 million new stroke cases each year and 7.5 million stroke survivors.[7,8] Stroke has had a significant impact on health care expenditures and the Chinese economy. In 2004, the average cost for stroke admission was ¥6,356 RMB ($1,271 AUD), which was two times greater than the annual income of rural residents of that year. The cost for stroke care by government-funded hospitals was ¥1.17 billion RMB in 2003 and ¥8.19 billion RMB in 2009, which is calculated as a 117% increase annually. It was reported that the annual cost of stroke care in China is approximately ¥40 billion RMB (in 2003), ten times higher than the care of cardiovascular diseases.[9,10]

Effective rehabilitation interventions initiated early after stroke can enhance the recovery process and minimise functional disability. Improved functional outcomes for patients also contribute to patient satisfaction and reduce potential costly long-term care expenditures. The primary goals of rehabilitation are to prevent complications, minimise impairments and maximise function.[11]

Certain post-stroke complications have a substantial effect on the final outcome of patients with stroke and often impede neurological recovery. Post-stroke complications can be summarised as the following main categories:

- Motor function complications: including muscle spasticity (an abnormal increase in muscle tone), joint contractures and shoulder problems.
- Cognitive and psychological complications: ranging from mild impairment of mental processes to severe dementia causing disability or psychological disorders such as depression and anxiety.
- Complications due to immobility: following a stroke, patients may have limited mobility which predisposes them to complications such as pressure sores and deep vein thrombosis.
- Infections: stroke patients are at risk of infections, particularly those affecting the chest and urinary tract.
- Disuse syndrome or misuse syndrome.

Of the motor function complications, shoulder-related complications are common and may negatively affect the upper limb's function and other rehabilitation outcomes, since good shoulder function is essential for successful transfers, maintaining balance, performing activities of daily living and for effective hand function.[12]

Definition of Post-stroke Shoulder Complications

Brief Introduction of the Shoulder Joint

The human shoulder is the most mobile joint in the body. This mobility provides the upper extremity with tremendous range of motion such as adduction, abduction, flexion, extension, internal rotation, external rotation, and 360° circumduction in the sagittal plane. Furthermore, the shoulder allows for scapular protraction, retraction, elevation and depression. This wide range of motion also makes the shoulder joint unstable. This instability is compensated for by rotator cuff muscles, tendons, ligaments and the glenoid labrum.[13]

The anatomy of the shoulder joint is different to most other joints in the body. The shoulder joint is a 'ball and socket' joint, where the head (the 'ball') of the humerus is contained in a thin articular capsule called the glenoid fossa (the 'socket'). This allows a wide range of movement in all directions, and relies on the surrounding muscles and ligaments to provide stability. Following a stroke, various changes such as decreased or increased muscle tone (spasticity) can lead to a range of shoulder complications. Three of the most common shoulder complications seen following stroke are shoulder subluxation, shoulder pain and shoulder-hand syndrome (SHS).[13]

Main Post-stroke Shoulder Complications

Shoulder Subluxation

Shoulder subluxation, or glenohumeral joint subluxation, is defined as a partial or incomplete dislocation that usually stems from changes in the mechanical integrity of the joint. For those post-stroke cases, shoulder subluxation is best explained as changes in the mechanical integrity of the glenohumeral joint causing a palpable gap between the acromion and humeral head.[12] During the initial period following a stroke, the hemiplegic arm is flaccid or hypotonic. In this stage the shoulder musculature, in particular the rotator cuff musculotendinous sleeve, cannot perform its function of maintaining the humeral head in the glenoid fossa, and there is a high risk of shoulder subluxation.[12] Over time, spasticity can lead to joint deformities.[14] Rotation of the shoulder musculature can pull the scapula downward, resulting in glenohumeral subluxation.[15]

It has been reported that shoulder subluxation occurs in 29–81% of patients with hemiplegia following stroke, due to muscle weakness or spasticity.[16] Shoulder subluxation is considered as an important source of shoulder pain,[16] and it possibly is associated with an increased incidence of SHS, also called complex regional pain syndrome (CRPS) of the upper limb.[17–19]

Shoulder Pain

Shoulder pain resulting from hemiplegia is a common clinical consequence of a focal cerebral insult resulting from a vascular lesion (i.e., haemorrhagic or ischaemic stroke). Hemiplegic shoulder pain may occur during movement of the shoulder joint, or even as spontaneous pain without movement. This can happen as early as two weeks post-stroke, but an onset time of 2–3 months post-stroke is more common.[12]

The development of hemiplegic shoulder pain is highly variable.[20] The presence of hemiplegic shoulder pain ranges from 16% to 72%,[21–24] and its prevalence is commonly estimated at between one-quarter and one-half of stroke patients.[21,24,25]

Shoulder-hand Syndrome

Pain following stroke which extends beyond the shoulder to involve the upper limb is classified as CRPS type I (more commonly known as SHS).[26] CRPS are neuropathic pain disorders which develop as an exaggerated response following nerve injury. Originally named reflex sympathetic dystrophy (RSD) and causalgia, the International Association for the Study of Pain (IASP) agreed on diagnostic criteria for RSD and causalgia, and subsequently renamed them CRPS types I and II, respectively. The key difference between types I and II relates to the identification of distinct nerve injury. In CRPS type II, a peripheral nerve lesion can be identified.[26] In CRPS type I, which is more common in stroke patients, a peripheral nerve lesion may not be detectable.[27]

Post-stroke upper limb CRPS (SHS) is prevalent in hemiplegic patients and can lead to significant medical complications.[26] It is characterized by numerous peripheral and central nervous system changes in the absence of obvious nerve injury. Peripheral changes include vasomotor tone with associated hand pain and swelling, exquisite tenderness or hyperaesthesia, protective immobility, trophic skin changes and vasomotor instability of the involved upper extremity. Central changes include a disruption of sensory cortical processing, disinhibiting of the motor cortex and disrupted body schema.[28,29]

Historically, a lack of consensus for diagnostic criteria for post-stroke SHS has resulted in significant variation in incidence estimates. Incidence has been described as low as 2%[30] and as high as 49%.[31]

Relationship between Subluxation, Pain and Shoulder-hand Syndrome

The post-stroke shoulder complications of subluxation, pain and SHS are closely correlated. Subluxation usually occurs during the acute stage of stroke. Decreased muscle tone and weakness following stroke can result in instability and decreased mobility in the glenohumeral joint, which can lead to glenohumeral subluxation.[4] In this stage, pain may develop along with the shoulder subluxation. Shoulder pain and SHS may develop one or two months later. Subluxation is considered to be one factor which contributes to shoulder pain, although the relationship between the two is not fully understood.[32] Also, subluxation is more common in patients who develop SHS,[33] which suggests that decreased mobility of the glenohumeral joint is involved in the development of SHS. This may be due to axillary nerve impingement and stretching of periarticular tissues.[34]

Table 1.1 summarises the main features of the three subtypes of shoulder complications.

Risk Factors of Post-stroke Shoulder Complications

Various risk factors have been identified which may predispose a patient to post-stroke shoulder complications. Risk factors include upper arm weakness, abnormal sensations and abnormal rheumatological exam,[35] stroke severity,[36] depression,[35] reduced arm function and supraspinatus tendon pathology.[37] Other risk factors reported by Harrison and Field[20] include female gender and older age at onset of stroke, previous medical history including use of alcohol and statins, depression and peripheral vascular disease, ischaemic stroke, thalamic or brainstem localisation, and factors following stroke such as spasticity and restricted arm movement.

Table 1.1   Main Post-stroke Shoulder Complications

Post-stroke Shoulder Complications — Subtypes	Main Features
Shoulder subluxation	During the initial period following a stroke, the shoulder musculature cannot perform its function of maintaining the humeral head in the glenoid fossa and there is a high risk of shoulder subluxation. It is defined as changes in the mechanical integrity of the glenohumeral joint causing a palpable gap between the acromion and humeral head. Shoulder subluxation is an important source of shoulder pain.
Shoulder pain	Common clinical consequence of a focal cerebral insult resulting from a vascular lesion. It may result in significant disability.
Shoulder-hand syndrome	Considered as complex regional pain syndrome type I, characterised by numerous peripheral changes including vasomotor tone with associated hand pain and swelling; exquisite tenderness or hyperaesthesia; protective immobility, trophic skin changes and vasomotor instability; and ventral changes including a disruption of sensory cortical processing, disinhibition of the motor cortex and disrupted body schema.

Shoulder subluxation is associated with the positioning of hemiplegia in the involved extremity during the initial flaccid stage of the condition. Improper positioning in bed, lack of support while the patient is in the upright position or pulling on the hemiplegic arm when transferring the patient all contribute to glenohumeral subluxation. Down and lateral subluxation commonly occur secondary to prolonged downward pull on the arm against which hypotonic muscles offer little resistance. The resulting mechanical effect is overstretching of the glenohumeral capsule (especially its superior aspect) and flaccid supraspinatus and deltoid muscles.[12] In addition, researchers have found a correlation between shoulder subluxation and rotator cuff injury, overstretching of ligaments and muscles (supraspinatus and deltoid), adhesive capsulitis, tendonitis, adhesions of the bicipital tendons, and rupture of ligaments.[38–43]

The cause of SHS is not yet fully understood. The onset and severity of SHS appear to be related with the aetiology of the stroke, the severity and recovery of motor deficit, spasticity and sensory disturbances. Another important aetiological factor is glenohumeral subluxation.[26] Some studies have indicated that cigarette smoking was strikingly present in patients and is statistically linked to SHS syndrome.[26]

Pathological Processes of Post-stroke Shoulder Complications

Shoulder subluxation is a common occurrence after stroke and can be due to muscle weakness or spasticity. Initially after stroke, one may experience a flaccid stage where the arm is limp, hangs down and has no movement. Soft tissue can become overstretched from the effects of gravity and improper handling of the arm. The theory to explain the development of post-stroke shoulder subluxation was developed in 1959.[16] During the flaccid stage, the trunk tends to lean or shorten toward the hemiplegic side, which causes the scapula to descend from its normal horizontal level. The trapezium and the serratus anterior also become flaccid, causing the scapula to rotate downward. Without normal tone, the rotator cuff can no longer maintain the integrity of the shoulder joint. These conditions contribute to a subluxing shoulder joint. During the spastic stage, the pectoralis major and minor, rhomboideus, elevator scapulae, and latissimus dorsi can become hypertonic, further rotating the scapula downward, causing shoulder subluxation.[16]

Several mechanisms of pain following stroke have been reported. Central mechanisms include thalamic lesions, cortical sensory abnormalities and maladaptive neuroplasticity, while peripheral mechanisms include inflammation and/or oedema, decreased muscle tone and limb hypoxia.[20] Increased adrenergic sensitivity and sympathetically maintained pain have also been identified as contributors to post-stroke pain, as have psychological factors such as depression, anxiety and heightened stress resulting from pain.[20] Many, or all, of these factors may interact to contribute to pain.

Understanding the pathogenesis of SHS (CRPS type I) in post-stroke patients is complex, as it is difficult to separate the pathophysiology of SHS from that related to the stroke event itself.[44] As outlined above, impaired movement of the glenohumeral joint is associated with development of SHS in post-stroke patients.[33] Trauma to the affected shoulder has been identified as the initiating factor for development of CRPS in post-stroke patients,[45] and post-mortem evidence of shoulder trauma was seen in patients with post-stroke SHS.[26] The severity of weakness and immobility and lower recovery status can also be a predictor of developing SHS.[46] The mechanisms which produce the broad range of symptoms reported in post-stroke SHS are not known.[44]

In CRPS, there is an exaggerated inflammatory response. Chemical mediators have been identified in the inflammatory soup around the primary afferent fibres that, through different processes, can induce hyper-excitability of the afferent fibres (peripheral sensitisation). It is hypothesised that a localised neurogenic inflammation is at the basis of the oedema, vasodilation and hyperhidrosis that are present in the initial phases of CRPS. The repeated discharge of the C-fibres causes an increased medullary excitability (central sensitisation). Another important factor is the reorganisation of the central nervous system, and in particular this appears to affect the primary somatosensory cortex. The central role of the sympathetic nerve is presently in doubt. However, it is thought that a subgroup of CRPS patients exists in whom a predominant factor is the hyperactivity of the sympathetic nervous system, and that it responds positively to sympathetic block.[26]

Diagnosis of Post-stroke Shoulder Complications

Shoulder Subluxation

In a shoulder subluxation, the humeral head slips out of the glenoid cavity as a result of weakness in the rotator cuff or a blow to the shoulder area. A subluxation can occur as one of three types: anterior (forward), posterior (backward), and inferior (downward). The difference between a shoulder subluxation and a shoulder dislocation is the fact that the humeral head pops back into its socket in the latter. The diagnosis of shoulder subluxation could be through clinical symptoms and functional testing.[16]

Patients with shoulder subluxations commonly present with pain in the shoulder region, loss of range of movement and a palpable gap between acromion and humeral head (this can be informally measured in finger-widths). A positive subluxation test (resistance is given, when the patient brings the arm to a throwing stance, in the internal rotation direction) could assist the diagnosis. Radiographic measurements are considered to be the most accurate way of evaluating the degree of subluxation.[16]

Shoulder Pain

The diagnosis of post-stroke shoulder pain can be achieved by a thorough clinical examination. Physical examination is important for diagnosis, as pain severity can be greater than self-reported pain. In fact, pain was identified through physical examination in up to 40% of patients who denied experiencing pain.[24] Physical signs of pain as sequelae to stroke included tenderness of the supraspinatus muscle or bicipital tendon, and a positive Neer sign.[24] The Neer test is a test for subacromial impingement, where the patient's arm is internally rotated and moved by the examiner through the full range of forward flexion or until pain is reported.

Further, the use of sonography may assist the diagnosis of hemiplegic shoulder pain. Shoulder pain is closely correlated to soft tissue injury in the shoulder, limitation of shoulder motion, sensory impairment, shoulder subluxation and spasticity. Musculoskeletal sonography is a convenient and inexpensive imaging tool for evaluating rotator cuff injuries among hemiplegic stroke patients. Main structural abnormalities can be found on the long head of the biceps tendon and supraspinatus tendon through shoulder sonography.[47,48]

Shoulder-hand Syndrome

The diagnosis of SHS in stroke patients appears more complex than in other diseases, since the paretic upper limb is frequently painful, oedematous, and displays altered heat and tactile sensitivity and slightly diastrophic skin within a non-use syndrome.[26] Therefore, the diagnosis of SHS should be based on clinical symptoms, and there are neither specific tests nor pathognomonic symptoms to identify this disease with certainty. The clinical features of SHS include:[26]

- Pain
    - Spontaneous;
    - Allodynia;
    - Hyperalgesia.
- Motor disturbances
    - Tremors;
    - Weakness;
    - Lack of muscular coordination;
    - Decreased range of motion (ROM);
    - Myoclonus;
    - Dystonia.
- Skin changes
    - Colour changes;
    - Pseudomotor abnormalities;
    - Temperature dysregulation;
    - Oedema/swelling;
    - Nail growth.
- Psychological distress
    - Anxiety;
    - Depression.

In addition to the clinical symptoms and signs, diagnostic tests may be used to support or assist confirmation of a diagnosis. Bone loss may be evident in late stage,[49,50] and skin thickening, soft tissue oedema and tissue enhancement with contrast material may be evident on magnetic resonance imaging.[51]

Management of Post-stroke Shoulder Complications

Preventing Subluxation and Pain

Prevention of shoulder pain is critical for post-stroke management.[52] Stabilisation of the shoulder joint after onset of motor weakness, whilst the musculature is flaccid, is important to avoid further injury. Physiotherapy starting with passive movement through the ROM should be initiated when the patient is medically stable.[53]

Proper positioning of the weak arm, as well as the use of arm slings where appropriate, can prevent the onset and reduce the progression of shoulder subluxation. Subluxation rarely resolves spontaneously;[54] also, currently there is no evidence that subluxation can be reduced after it has occurred, so prevention is essential.[55] Management of subluxation consists of strategies to prevent it worsening. Interventions aimed at reducing trauma to the shoulder, such as educating all staff, carers and stroke survivors, should prevent the occurrence of shoulder subluxation and pain resulting from the weakness. Such education may include strategies to care for the shoulder during manual handling and transfers and advice regarding positioning.[55]

Preventing subluxation should help to prevent pain. For people with severe weakness who are at risk of developing shoulder pain, management may include shoulder strapping and educating staff, carers and people with stroke about preventing trauma.[55]

Management of Pain

Options for pain management once the full pain syndrome has developed include stabilisation using shoulder slings and strapping, and lap boards or arm troughs in wheelchairs if required. Initiation of pain management with medication should use a stepped approach, with simple analgesics and non-steroidal anti-inflammatories as first-line therapy.[52] For patients with hypertonicity, anti-spasmodic agents may be used in combination with physiotherapy.[56]

Transcutaneous neuromuscular electrical stimulation (TENS), which activates myelinated sensory fibres and disrupts transmission of pain signals of unmyelinated C-fibres,[57] may be considered. Isometric electrical strength of the shoulder girdle may be maintained through the use of functional electrical stimulation of the supraspinatus and posterior deltoid muscles.[58] This has been shown to improve the range of motion and arm function and reduce pain.[59]

Corticosteroid injection into the glenohumeral joint or subacromial space has been used clinically to treat shoulder pain. Currently there is limited evidence to confirm the effects.[4] Botulinum toxin injections have shown improvement and resolution of shoulder pain.[60] Suprascapular nerve blocks may be effective in reducing shoulder pain through a reduction of both nociceptive and neuropathic pain mechanisms.[4] Where pain is not controlled with the treatment options highlighted above, surgery may be considered. Surgery can be used to repair rotator cuff tears, for muscle tendon contractures and to promote mobilisation of the scapular.[20]

In addition, it has been suggested that acupuncture, in combination with standard therapeutic exercise, may be a safe and effective adjuvant for treatment of hemiplegic shoulder pain.[4] Massage and acupressure have also been evaluated by clinical research; currently there is insufficient evidence to support the benefit of these compared to conventional treatment in post-stroke shoulder pain.[61]

Management of Swelling of Extremity

People who are upright (standing or sitting) with their arm hanging and immobile as result of a weakness are at risk of developing swelling of the hand. Management of swelling includes the use of dynamic pressure garments, electrical stimulation and elevation of the limb when resting — all these can be considered for preventing or reducing swelling.[55]

Management of Shoulder-hand Syndrome

Since the cause of CRPS has not yet been clearly understood, treatment of post-stroke SHS may include a range of approaches. Treatment options include pharmacological, regional anaesthesia, neuromodulation, sympathectomy, psychotherapy and non-pharmacological options.[26] Treatment for SHS is most effective when started early. In such cases, improvement and even remission are possible. The primary aims of treatment are to reduce pain, to restore arm function and to maintain mobility of the shoulder joint.[26] Paramount to care is ensuring mobilisation and strengthening of the affected arm, desensitisation techniques and oedema control; this interdisciplinary approach involves both occupational and physical therapists.[26]

Prevention of joint injury may reduce the incidence of SHS. Passive movement by therapists and restriction of passive movement by patients have been successful in preventing SHS in some patients.[62] For management of pain, nerve blocks at the level of the stellate ganglion can be considered if pain is sympathetically mediated.[63] Desensitisation, including increasing levels of sensory stimulation or contrast baths with increasing temperature differences, may help to return normal processing of sensory stimuli.[64] Non-pharmacological therapies may provide some benefit. Mirror therapy, where patients watch the movement of the unaffected limb in a mirror, has been shown to improve kinaesthetic sensations of movement in amputees and post-stroke hemiparesis.[65] Such activity is thought to stimulate the premotor cortex to assist with motor rehabilitation, through its influence on bilateral movement control and connections between visual input and premotor areas.[65] It is well understood that the inter-relationship between physical and psychosocial factors is important in pain. The evidence is inconclusive as to whether pre-morbid psychological symptoms contribute to the development of SHS, but SHS has been showed to impair psychological well-being.[66] Treatment directed at improving psychological symptoms is important in managing pain.[66,67]

Pharmacological treatments for SHS are outlined in various guidelines and reviews.[68–71] Recommended treatments include anticonvulsants such as gabapentin and carbamazepine, and tricyclic antidepressants. Information from two systematic reviews showed tricyclic antidepressants to be effective regardless of cause of neuropathic pain,[71] and thus can be considered for pain management in post-stroke central pain. Due to the pathogenesis of inflammation following stroke, treatments which target inflammation may also be effective in controlling post-stroke pain. Corticosteroids have been shown to be more effective than piroxicam in improving pain in post-stroke SHS,[72] while a short course of oral glucocorticoids provided significant pain relief in a small clinical trial of hemiplegic patients with SHS.[73]

Table 1.2 summarises the definition, diagnosis and management of post-stroke shoulder complications.

Table 1.2 Summary of Post-stroke Shoulder Complications: Definition, Diagnosis and Management

Definition	• Shoulder subluxation is defined as a partial or incomplete dislocation that usually stems from changes in the mechanical integrity of the joint. • Post-stroke pain is a frequently seen complication after stroke, and can be caused by central and peripheral mechanisms, autonomic input and psychological factors. • Shoulder-hand syndrome (complex regional pain syndrome type I) is a neuropathic pain disorder that develops as an exaggerated response to a traumatic lesion or nerve damage.
Diagnosis	• Shoulder subluxation: pain in the shoulder region, loss of range of movement and palpable gap between acromion and humeral head, a positive subluxation test, and radiographic measurements. • Shoulder pain: a thorough clinical examination. • Shoulder-hand syndrome (complex regional pain syndrome): the diagnosis of shoulder-hand syndrome is essentially clinical. Main clinical features are pain, motor disturbances, skin changes and possible psychological distress.
Management	• Shoulder subluxations: proper positioning, slings, strapping and education. • Shoulder pain: proper positioning, slings, strapping, education, analgesics and non-steroidal anti-inflammation medications, anti-spasmodic agents, skin surface electrical stimulation, corticosteroid injection, botulinum toxin injections, suprascapular nerve blocks and surgery. • Shoulder-hand syndrome: non-pharmacological, pharmacological with psychotherapy, regional anaesthesia, neuromodulation and sympathectomy.

Prognosis of Post-stroke Shoulder Complications

Shoulder subluxation or loosening of the shoulder joint, caused by the weight and pressure of a weak arm, occurs in the early stage after stroke. If untreated, shoulder subluxation can progress to cause pain and SHS.

Upon the development of SHS, the affected limb can become cold and pale and undergo skin and nail changes as well as muscle spasms and tightening. Once these changes occur, the condition is often irreversible. CRPS occasionally may spread from its source to elsewhere in the body, such as the opposite limb. The pain may be worsened by emotional stress.

References

1. Recommendations on stroke prevention, diagnosis, and therapy. Report of the WHO Task Force on Stroke and Other Cerebrovascular Disorders. (1989) *Stroke* **20**(10): 1407–1431.
2. World Health Organization. (2014) Global status report on noncommunicable diseases. Available from: http://www.who.int/nmh/publications/ncd-status-report-2014/en/.
3. American Heart Association. (2004) Heart and stroke statistical update — 2005.
4. Winstein CJ, Stein J, Arena R, *et al.* (2016) Guidelines for adult stroke rehabilitation and recovery: A guideline for healthcare professionals from the American Heart Association/American Stroke Association. American Heart Association Stroke Council, Council on Cardiovascular and Stroke Nursing, Council on Clinical Cardiology, and Council on Quality of Care and Outcomes Research. *Stroke* **47**(6): e98–e169.
5. Australian Institute of Health and Welfare. (2012) Australia's health 2012. Australia's health series no.13. Cat. no. AUS 156. Available from: https://www.aihw.gov.au.
6. National Stroke Foundation. (2013) The economic impact of stroke in Australia. Available from: file://rmit.internal/USRHome/el6/E77936/Downloads/Final-Deloitte-Stroke-Report-14-Mar-13%20(3).pdf.
7. Johnston SC, Mendis S, Mathers CD. (2009) Global variation in stroke burden and mortality: Estimates from monitoring, surveillance, and modelling. *Lancet Neurol* **8**(4): 345–354.
8. 陈竺. (2008) 全国样本地区死亡率水平与死亡原因. 全国第三次死因回顾抽样调查报告. 北京: 中国协和医科大学出版社.

9. 胡善联, 龚向光. (2003) 中国缺血性脑卒中的疾病经济负担. 中国卫生经济 **22**(12): 18–20.

10. 中华人民共和国卫生部. (2010) 年度中国卫生保健统计. 北京: 中国协和医科大学出版社.

11. Duncan PW, Zorowitz R, Bates B, *et al.* (2005) Management of adult stroke rehabilitation care: A clinical practice guideline. *Stroke* **36**(9): e100–e143.

12. Mehta S, Teasull R, Foley N. (last updated 2018) Evidence-based review of stroke rehabilitation: Painful hemiplegic shoulder. Available from: http://www.ebrsr.com/evidence-review/11-hemiplegic-shoulder-pain-complex-regional-pain-syndrome.

13. Moore KL, Agur AMR, eds. (2007) *Upper Limb: Essential Clinical Anatomy*, 3rd ed. Lippincott Williams & Wilkins, Philadelphia, pp. 407–490.

14. Patel AT. (2010) Early diagnosis of post-stroke spasticity and treatment options. *US Neurol* **5**(2): 47–51.

15. Cailliet R. (1980) *The Shoulder in Hemiplegia*, 3rd ed. FA Davis Co, Philadelphia, pp. 78–86.

16. Paci M, Nannetti L, Rinaldi LA. (2005) Glenohumeral subluxation in hemiplegia: An overview. *J Rehabil Res Dev* **42**(4): 557–568.

17. Dursun E, Dursun N, Ural CE, Cakci A. (2000) Glenohumeral joint subluxation and reflex sympathetic dystrophy in hemiplegic patients. *Arch Phys Med Rehabil* **81**: 944–946.

18. Tepperman PS, Greyson ND, Hilbert L, *et al.* (1984) Reflex sympathetic dystrophy in hemiplegia. *Arch Phys Med Rehabil* **65**: 442–447.

19. Chang JJ, Tsau JC, Lin YT. (1995) Predictors of shoulder subluxation in stroke patients. *Kaohsiung J Med Sci* **11**: 250–256.

20. Harrison RA, Field TS. (2015) Post stroke pain: Identification, assessment, and therapy. *Cerebrovasc Dis* **39**(3–4): 190–201.

21. Gamble GE, Barberan E, Bowsher D, *et al.* (2000) Post stroke shoulder pain: More common than previously realized. *Eur J Pain* **4**: 313–315.

22. Roy CW, Sands MR, Hill LD. (1994) Shoulder pain in acutely admitted hemiplegics. *Clin Rehabil* **8**: 334–340.

23. Dromerick A, Reding M. (1994) Medical and neurological complications during inpatient stroke rehabilitation. *Stroke* **25**: 358–361.

24. Dromerick AW, Edwards DF, Kumar A. (2008) Hemiplegic shoulder pain syndrome: Frequency and characteristics during inpatient stroke rehabilitation. *Arch Phys Med Rehabil* **89**: 1589–1593.

25. Lindgren I, Jönsson AC, Norrving B, Lindgren A. (2007) Shoulder pain after stroke: A prospective population-based study. *Stroke* **38**: 343–348.

26. Pertoldi S, Di Benedetto P. (2005) Shoulder-hand syndrome after stroke. A complex regional pain syndrome. *Eura Medicophys* **41**(4): 283–292.

27. Weber M, Birklein F. (2001) Complex regional pain syndrome: An actual survey. *Expert Rev Neurother* **1**(1): 100–109.

28. Moseley GL. (2004) Graded motor imagery is effective for long-standing complex regional pain syndrome: A randomised controlled trial. *Pain* **108**(1–2): 192–198.

29. Moseley GL. (2006) Graded motor imagery for pathologic pain: A randomized controlled trial. *Neurology* **67**(12): 2129–2134.

30. McLean DE. (2004) Medical complications experienced by a cohort of stroke survivors during inpatient, tertiary-level stroke rehabilitation. *Arch Phys Med Rehabil* **85**: 466–469.

31. Kocabas H, Levendoglu F, Ozerbil OM, Yuruten B. (2007) Complex regional pain syndrome in stroke patients. *Int J Rehabil Res* **30**: 33–38.

32. Paci M, Nannetti L, Taiti P, *et al.* (2007) Shoulder subluxation after stroke: Relationships with pain and motor recovery. *Physiother Res Int* **12**: 95–104.

33. Dursun E, Dursun N, Ural CE, Cakci A. (2000) Glenohumeral joint subluxation and reflex sympathetic dystrophy in hemiplegic patients. *Arch Phys Med Rehabil* **81**: 944–946.

34. Ring H, Leillen B, Server S, *et al.* (1985) Temporal changes in electrophysiological, clinical and radiological parameters in the hemiplegic's shoulder. *Scand J Rehabil Med Suppl* **12**: 124–127.

35. Gamble GE, Barberan E, Laasch HU, *et al.* (2002) Poststroke shoulder pain: A prospective study of the association and risk factors in 152 patients from a consecutive cohort of 205 patients presenting with stroke. *Eur J Pain* **6**(6): 467–474.

36. Rajaratnam BS, Venketasubramanian N, Kumar PV, *et al.* (2007) Predictability of simple clinical tests to identify shoulder pain after stroke. *Arch Phys Med Rehabil.* **88**: 1016–1021.

37. Kim YH, Jung SJ, Yang EJ, Paik NJ. (2014) Clinical and sonographic risk factors for hemiplegic shoulder pain: A longitudinal observational study. *J Rehabil Med* **46**(1): 81–87.

38. Najenson T, Yacubovich E, Pikielni SS. (1971) Rotator cuff injury in shoulder joints in hemiplegic patients. *Scand J Rehabil Med* **3**: 131–137.

39. Chino N. Electrophysiological investigation on shoulder subluxation in hemiplegics. *Scand J Rehabil Med* (1981) **13**: 17–21.

40. Shahani BT, Kelly EB, Glasse S. (1981) Hemiplegic shoulder subluxation. *Arch Phys Med Rehabil* **62**: 17–21.
41. Griffin JW. (1986) Hemiplegic shoulder pain. *Phys Ther* **66**: 1884–1893.
42. Hakuno A, Sahika H, Ohkawa T, Itoh R. (1984) Arthrographic findings in hemiplegic shoulders. *Arch Phys Med Rehabil* **65**: 706–711.
43. Jensen EM. (1980) The hemiplegic shoulder. *Scand J Rehabil Med Suppl* **7**: 113–119.
44. Chae J. (2010) Poststroke complex regional pain syndrome. *Top Stroke Rehabil* **17**: 151–162.
45. Geurts AC, Visschers BA, Van Limbeek J, Ribbers GM. (2000) Systematic review of aetiology and treatment of post-stroke hand oedema and shoulder-hand syndrome. *Scand J Rehabil Med* **32**(1): 4–10.
46. Gokkaya NK, Aras M, Yesiltepe E, Koseoglu F. (2006) Reflex sympathetic dystrophy in hemiplegia. *Int J Rehabil Res* **29**: 275–279.
47. Huang YC, Liang PJ, Pong YP, *et al.* (2010) Physical findings and sonography of hemiplegic shoulder in patients after acute stroke during rehabilitation. *J Rehabil Med* **42**(1): 21–26.
48. Pong YP, Wang LY, Wang L, *et al.* (2009) Sonography of the shoulder in hemiplegic patients undergoing rehabilitation after a recent stroke. *J Clin Ultrasound* **37**(4): 199–205.
49. Kozin F, Genant HK, Bekerman C, McCarty DJ. (1976) The reflex sympathetic dystrophy syndrome. II. Roentgenographic and scintigraphic evidence of bilaterality and of periarticular accentuation. *Am J Med* **60**: 332–338.
50. Sambrook P, Champion GD. (1990) Reflex sympathetic dystrophy; characteristic changes in bone on CT scan. *J Rheumatol* **17**: 1425–1426.
51. Schweitzer ME, Mandel S, Schwartzman RJ, *et al.* (1995) Reflex sympathetic dystrophy revisited: MR imaging findings before and after infusion of contrast material. *Radiology* **195**: 211–214.
52. Dawson AS, Knox J, McClure A, *et al.* (2013) Stroke Rehabilitation Best Practices Writing Group: Management of shoulder pain following stroke. In: Lindsay MP, Gubitz G, Bayley M, Phillips S (eds), *Canadian Best Practice Recommendations for Stroke Care*. Heart and Stroke Foundation and the Canadian Stroke Network, Ottawa, Ontario, pp. 47–50.
53. Vasudevan JM, Browne BJ. (2014) Hemiplegic shoulder pain: An approach to diagnosis and management. *Phys Med Rehabil Clin N Am* **25**: 411–437.
54. Zorowitz RD. (2001) Recovery patterns of shoulder subluxation after stroke: A six-month follow up study. *Top Stroke Rehabil* **8**: 1–9.

55. The Stroke Foundation. (2010) Clinical guidelines for stroke management. Available from: https://www.pedro.org.au/wp-content/uploads/CPG_stroke.pdf.
56. Van Ouwenaller C, Laplace PM, Chantraine A. (1986) Painful shoulder in hemiplegia. *Arch Phys Med Rehabil* **67**: 23–26.
57. Garrison DW, Foreman RD. (1994) Decreased activity of spontaneous and noxiously evoked dorsal horn cells during transcutaneous electrical nerve stimulation (TENS). *Pain* **58**: 309–315.
58. Linn SL, Granat MH, Lees KR. (1999) Prevention of shoulder subluxation after stroke with electrical stimulation. *Stroke* **30**: 963–968.
59. Faghri PD, Rodgers MM, Glaser RM, *et al.* (1994) The effects of functional electrical stimulation on shoulder subluxation, arm function recovery, and shoulder pain in hemiplegic stroke patients. *Arch Phys Med Rehabil* **75**: 73–79.
60. Bhakta BB, Cozens JA, Bamford JM, Chamberlain MA. (1996) Use of botulinum toxin in stroke patients with severe upper limb spasticity. *J Neurol Neurosurg Psychiatry* **61**: 30–35.
61. Scottish Intercollegiate Guidelines Network. (2010) Management of patients with stroke: Rehabilitation, prevention and management of complications, and discharge planning: A national clinical guideline. Available from: http://www.sign.ac.uk/assets/sign118.pdf.
62. Kondo I, Hosokawa K, Soma M. (2001) Protocol to prevent shoulder hand syndrome after stroke. *Arch Phys Med Rehabil* **82**: 1619–1623.
63. Wasner G, Schattschneider J, Binder A, Baron R. (2003) Complex regional pain syndrome: Diagnostic, mechanisms, CNS involvement and therapy. *Spinal Cord* **41**: 61–75.
64. Harden RN. (2001) Complex regional pain syndrome. *Br J Anaesth* **87**: 99–106.
65. Altschuler EL, Wisdom SB, Stone L, *et al.* (1999) Rehabilitation of hemiparesis after stroke with a mirror: Early recanalisation in acute ischaemic stroke saves tissue at risk defined by MRI. *Lancet* **353**: 2036–2037.
66. Lohnberg JA, Altmaier EM. (2013) A review of psychosocial factors in complex regional pain syndrome. *J Clin Psychol Med Settings* **20**: 247–254.
67. Gierthmuhlen J, Binder A, Baron R. (2014) Mechanism-based treatment in complex regional pain syndromes. *Nat Rev Neurol* **10**: 518–528.
68. Finnerup NB, Attal N, Haroutounian S, *et al.* (2015) Pharmacotherapy for neuropathic pain in adults: A systematic review and meta-analysis. *Lancet Neurol* **14**(2): 162–173.

69. Attal N, Cruccu G, Baron R, *et al.* (2010) European Federation of Neurological Societies. EFNS guidelines on the pharmacological treatment of neuropathic pain: 2010 revision. *Eur J Neurol* **17**(9): 1113–e88.
70. Haanpää M, Attal N, Backonja M, *et al.* (2011) NeuPSIG guidelines on neuropathic pain assessment. *Pain* **152**(1): 14–27.
71. Moulin DE, Clark AJ, Gilron I, *et al.* (2007) Canadian Pain Society. Pharmacological management of chronic neuropathic pain: Consensus statement and guidelines from the Canadian Pain Society. *Pain Res Manag* **12**(1): 13–21.
72. Kalita J, Vajpayee A, Misra UK. (2006) Comparison of prednisolone with piroxicam in complex regional pain syndrome following stroke: A randomized controlled trial. *QJM* **99**: 89–95.
73. Braus DF, Krauss JK, Strobel J. (1994) The shoulder-hand syndrome after stroke: A prospective clinical trial. *Ann Neurol* **36**: 728–733.

2

Post-stroke Shoulder Complications in Chinese Medicine

OVERVIEW

This chapter describes the aetiology, pathogenesis, syndrome differentiation and treatments recommended in key Chinese medicine clinical textbooks and guidelines. In Chinese medicine, post-stroke shoulder complications are considered as the results of disordered *qi* 气 and Blood after stroke. Syndrome differentiation of post-stroke shoulder dysfunction is seldom seen in the present guidelines, literature or textbooks. The most common syndrome differentiation used in Chinese herbal medicine treatments is meridian stroke 中经络. Acupuncture and *tuina* 推拿 therapy applied on the local area are also recommended.

Introduction

Shoulder subluxation, shoulder pain and shoulder-hand syndrome are common post-stroke complications. They are usually seen as shoulder and upper limb symptoms of post-stroke motor function impairment, and may negatively affect rehabilitation outcomes of upper limb functions. In Chinese medicine (CM) classical literature, these complications have not been recorded as a specific clinical condition.

The terminologies used in classical literature referring to stroke and its motor function complications include *pu ji* 仆击, *bo jue* 薄厥, *pian ku* 偏枯, *pian feng* 偏风, *feng fei* 风痱, and *ban shen bu sui* 半身不遂. For instance, the Plain Questions-Discourse on Wind

(*Su Wen* 素问 • 风论, Chapter 42) states: 'When the Wind strikes the transporting (*shu* 俞) points of the five *zang* 脏 and six *fu* 腑, this causes Wind of the *zang fu* 脏腑. In each case it enters through the respective door. Where Wind attacks, unilateral Wind results.' The Miraculous Pivot-Discussion on the Five Sections in Needling and Comments on the Genuine Qi and Pathogenic Factors (*Lingshu* 灵枢 • 刺节真邪篇, Chapter 75) states: 'When the deficient pathogenic factor attacks the upper part of the body, it may penetrate deeply, lodging internally in the nutrient *qi* 营气 and defensive *qi* 卫气. Once the nutrient *qi* 营气 and defensive *qi* 卫气 become debilitated, the genuine *qi* 真气 recedes and the pathogenic *qi* 气 alone remains in the body, causing *pian ku* 偏枯.' It is stated in the A-B Classic of Acupuncture and Moxibustion — The Contraction of Disease by Yang Producing Wind (*Zhen Jiu Jia Yi Jing* 针灸甲乙经, Volume Ten, Chapter 2 (Part 2)): '*Pian ku* 偏枯 means half of the body is unmovable and painful. *Pian ku* 偏枯 causes pains in the arm and wrist which sometimes flex and cannot extend. There are pains in the shoulders and elbows causing difficulty with flexion and extension, inability of the hands to lift weights, and hypertonicity of the wrists.' Shoulder dysfunction often occurs after stroke and is characterised by localised pain in the muscles and joints, swelling, and difficulty with flexion and extension. Though these manifestations are seemingly similar to those of *bi syndrome* 痹证 in CM, the aetiology and pathogenesis behind them are very close to those of stroke. These manifestations show the fundamental pathogenesis of stroke on localised body parts.

Aetiology and Pathogenesis

Stroke can be caused by the dysfunction of *zang fu* 脏腑, vital *qi* 正气 deficiency, emotional disturbances, overwork, internal injuries, irregular diet and sudden climate changes.[1] The root (*ben* 本) of the condition is deficient and the tip (*biao* 标) is excessive; the upper part of the body is with excess syndrome and the lower with deficiency. There is *yin* 阴 deficiency of the Liver and Kidney, deficiency of *qi* 气 and Blood, Wind and fire interacting and attacking, sever phlegm-dampness obstruction, reversed *qi* 气 flow, and Blood stasis. 'Vital *qi* 正气 deficiency causing pathogenic-*qi* 邪气 stroke' is elaborated in the Internal Classic (*Huang Di Nei Jing* 黄帝内经): 'Pulse at *cun kou* 寸口 is floating and tight. Tense pulse indicates existence of pathogenic cold; floating pulse signifies a case of a deficient nature. Pathogenic cold and deficiency coexist. Pathogenic cold first rests on the skin. Floating pulse indicates Blood deficiency with collaterals void and defenseless, allowing pathogenic factors to circulate throughout the body, sometimes on the left side, sometimes on the right. When either side of the body is affected, muscles and meridians become loose. By comparison, the side which is not affected seems tense, and distortion of the mouth and eyes takes place on this side, with hemiplegia.' This statement explains the pathogenesis of stroke: 'Collaterals are void and defenseless, allowing pathogenic factors to circulate throughout the body.'

Shoulder dysfunction can be attributed to disordered *qi* 气 and Blood after stroke. Phlegm and static Blood accumulate in the diseased side of the limbs, blocking meridians and collaterals, which results in hemilateral withering of limbs. *Qi* 气 stagnation and Blood stasis obstruct the Blood vessels, which hinders the free flow of *qi* 气 and Blood and causes pain. Phlegm is sticky and stagnant; static Blood, being heavy and turbid, does not circulate properly; *qi* 气 is deficient and unable to activate the movement of fluids and Blood. The failure of stagnant Blood flowing freely leads to water retention with swelling and distention. Deficiency of *qi* 气 and Blood causes slowed Blood flow which leads to stasis; as a result, malnourishment of the tendons and vessels occurs, which causes flexion and spasm. The fundamental etiology and pathogenesis of post-stroke shoulder dysfunction can be summarized as *qi* 气 deficiency and Blood stasis causing obstruction of meridians and collaterals. The condition is deficient in the root (*ben* 本) and excessive in the tip (*biao* 标).

Syndrome Differentiation and Treatments

The location, severity, and pathogenic changes of stroke in different patients may vary. Importance should be attached to the identification of meridian stroke 中经络 and *zang fu* stroke 中脏腑, stages, and pathogenic changes. Acute stroke can be classified into two categories: Meridian stroke 中经络 and *zang fu* stroke 中脏腑. Meridian stroke 中经络 is characterised by hemiplegia, hemilateral numbness, distortion of the mouth and tongue, and difficult speaking.[1] Delirium is often an associated symptom of *zang fu* stroke 中脏腑. Stroke can be divided into three stages: acute, convalescent, and sequela. Post-stroke shoulder dysfunction is commonly seen in the convalescent and sequela stages. In the acute stage, most cases are meridian stroke 中经络 and the symptoms are mild in most patients who have no obvious problems with consciousness. The clinical manifestations include hemiplegia, shoulder joint swelling, distention, pain, difficulty with flexion and extension, with/without distortion of the mouth and tongue, and difficult speaking, etc.

The root (*ben* 本) of this condition is deficient and the tip (*biao* 标) is excessive. Though there is deficiency of vital *qi* 正气 in the acute stage, the tip (*biao* 标) is excessive for Wind, fire, phlegm, and stasis. Therefore, the treatment principles are pacifying the Liver and extinguishing Wind, clearing heat and scouring phlegm, resolving phlegm and unblocking *fu* 腑 organs, activating Blood and freeing the collateral vessels. In the convalescent and sequela stages, the syndrome is, mostly, combination of deficiency and excess syndromes. The treatment principles are reinforcing vital *qi* 正气 and eliminating pathogenic factors. Chinese herbal medicine (CHM) formulas for tonifying *qi* 气 and activating Blood, nourishing *yin* 阴 and freeing the collateral vessels, in combination with acupuncture, moxibustion, massage and other rehabilitating therapies, are often used to treat the disease.

Clarified syndrome differentiation of post-stroke shoulder dysfunction is seldom seen in the guidelines, literature or textbooks. The regularly applied syndrome differentiation in clinical practice is that of meridian stroke 中经络. The following syndrome differentiation and formulas are summarised from textbooks and clinical guidelines; these are *Chinese Medicine Internal Medicine* (中医内科学),[1] *Evidence-based Guidelines of Clinical Practice in Chinese Medicine Internal Medicine* (中医循证临床实践指南—中医内科)[2] and *Clinical*

Guidelines of Common Diseases in Chinese Medicine Internal Medicine (中医内科常见病诊疗指南),[3,4] while the reference for specific ingredients of formulas is *Zhong Yi Fang Ji Da Ci Dian* (中医方剂大辞典).[5]

Syndrome of Wind-fire Uprising 风火上扰证

Clinical manifestations: Hemiplegia, facial palsy, difficulty speaking or aphasia, hemilateral numbness, unfixed shoulder pain, dizziness, headaches, red complexion, red eyes, bitter taste in the mouth, dry throat, agitation, irritability, dark urine, dry stools, crimson tongue body, yellow, greasy and dry tongue coating, and string-like and rapid pulse.

Treatment principle: Calming the Liver to suppress *yang* 阳, and clearing heat to eliminate Wind.

Formula: Modified *Tian ma gou teng yin* 天麻钩藤饮加减.[1-4]

Herbs: *Tian ma* 天麻, *gou teng* 钩藤, *shi jue ming* 石决明, *chuan niu xi* 川牛膝, *du zhong* 杜仲, *sang ji sheng* 桑寄生, *huang qin* 黄芩, *zhi zi* 栀子, *yi mu cao* 益母草, *ye jiao teng* 夜交藤 and *fu shen* 茯神.

Analysis of formula: *Tian ma* 天麻 and *gou teng* 钩藤 calm the Liver and eliminate Wind; *shi jue ming* 石决明 calms the Liver and suppresses *yang* 阳; *chuan niu xi* 川牛膝 brings Blood downward; *huang qin* 黄芩 and *zhi zi* 栀子 clear the Liver and purge fire; *du zhong* 杜仲 and *sang ji sheng* 桑寄生 tonify and replenish the Liver and Kidney; *fu shen* 茯神 and *ye jiao teng* 夜交藤 tonify Blood and calm the mind; *yi mu cao* 益母草 activates Blood and induces diuresis. They are combined to suppress *yang* 阳 by calming the Liver, and to tonify and replenish the Liver and Kidney.

Syndrome of Wind-phlegm Obstructing the Collaterals 风痰阻络证

Clinical manifestations: Hemiplegia, hypertonicity of the limbs, facial palsy, difficulty speaking or aphasia, hemilateral numbness, shoulder swelling and pain which are relieved by warmth, dizziness, profuse and sticky phlegm, dark tongue, thin/greasy and white tongue coating, slippery and string-like pulse.

Treatment principle: Eliminating Wind, reducing phlegm, activating Blood and unblocking the collaterals.

Formula: Modified *hua tan tong luo tang* 化痰通络汤加减.[1-4]

Herbs: *Fa ban xia* 法半夏, *bai zhu* 白术, *tian ma* 天麻, *dan nan xing* 胆南星, *dan shen* 丹参, *xiang fu* 香附 and *jiu da huang* 酒大黄.

Analysis of formula: *Fa ban xia* 法半夏 and *bai zhu* 白术 dry dampness to strengthen the Spleen; *tian ma* 天麻 calms the Liver and eliminates Wind; *dan nan xing* 胆南星 clears heat and reduces phlegm; *xiang fu* 香附 soothes the Liver and regulates *qi* 气; *dan shen* 丹参 activates Blood and reduces phlegm; *jiu da huang* 酒大黄 unblocks *fu* 腑 organs. They are combined to reduce phlegm, eliminate Wind and unblock the collaterals.

Syndrome of Phlegm Heat and Excess in the *Fu* Organ 痰热腑实证

Clinical manifestations: Hemiplegia, stiffness and spasms of limbs, hemilateral numbness, shoulder swelling and burning pain, difficulty speaking, facial palsy, abdominal distension, dry stools, constipation, headaches, dizziness, expectoration/profuse phlegm, red tongue with yellow and greasy/dry tongue coating, and string-like/large and slippery pulse.

Treatment principle: Reducing phlegm and clearing the *fu* 腑 organ.

Formula: Modified *Xing lou cheng qi tang* 星蒌承气汤.[1-4]

Herbs: *Gua lou* 瓜蒌, *dan nan xing* 胆南星, *da huang* 大黄 and *mang xiao* 芒硝.

Analysis of formula: *Gua lou* 瓜蒌 and *dan nan xing* 胆南星 clear heat and reduce phlegm; *da huang* 大黄 and *mang xiao* 芒硝 clear the stomach and intestines, unblock *fu* 腑 organ, and purge heat. The modification of dosage or exclusion of *da huang* 大黄 and *mang xiao*

芒硝, in consideration of the condition and constitution of the patients, is sometimes needed to avoid damaging vital *qi* 正气.

Syndrome of *Qi* Deficiency with Blood Stasis 气虚血瘀证

Clinical manifestations: Hemiplegia, reduced muscular tension of affected limbs, hemilateral numbness, should pain which shows increased piercing pain at night and with local stagnated vessels, swelling and distension of feet and hands, facial palsy, difficulty speaking, whitish complexion, shortness of breath, lack of strength, sialorrhea, palpitation, loose stools, dark tongue with white and greasy coating, and deep and thin pulse. They often occur in the convalescent and sequela stages, sometimes in the acute stage.

Treatment principle: Tonifying *qi* 气 and activating Blood.

Formula: Modified *Bu yang huan wu tang* 补阳还五汤加减.[1-4]

Herbs: *Huang qi* 黄芪, *dang gui* 当归, *tao ren* 桃仁, *hong hua* 红花, *chi shao* 赤芍, *chuang xiong* 川芎 and *di long* 地龙.

Analysis of formula: *Huang qi* 黄芪 is largely applied to tonify *qi* 气, which helps promote Blood flow and eliminate stasis without damaging vital *qi* 正气; *dang gui* 当归, *tao ren* 桃仁, *hong hua* 红花, *chi shao* 赤芍, *chuang xiong* 川芎 and *di long* 地龙 work together to activate Blood, reduce phlegm and unblock the collaterals.

Syndrome of *Yin* Deficiency with Stirring Wind 阴虚风动证

Clinical manifestations: Hemiplegia, hemilateral numbness, shoulder pain, reduced muscle tone, spasms, weakness and inability to lift, facial palsy, difficulty speaking, dizziness, tinnitus, feverishness in chest, palms and soles, dry throat and mouth, red and emaciated tongue with little/ no tongue coating, and fine and rapid pulse. These are usually seen in the convalescent and sequela stages, sometimes in the acute stage.

Treatment principle: Tonifying *yin* 阴, suppressing *yang* 阳, calming the Liver and eliminating Wind.

Formula: Modified *Zhen gan xi feng tang* 镇肝熄风汤加减.[1-3]

Herbs: *Niu xi* 牛膝, *sheng long gu* 生龙骨, *sheng mu li* 生牡蛎, *dai zhe shi* 代赭石, *gui ban* 龟板, *bai shao* 白芍, *xuan shen* 玄参, *tian men dong* 天门冬, *chuan lian zi* 川楝子, *mai ya* 麦芽, *yin chen* 茵陈 and *gan cao* 甘草.

Analysis of formula: *Sheng long gu* 生龙骨, *sheng mu li* 生牡蛎 and *dai zhe shi* 代赭石 calm the Liver to suppress *yang* 阳; *gui ban* 龟板, *bai shao* 白芍, *xuan shen* 玄参 and *tian men dong* 天门冬 enrich *yin* 阴 and suppress *yang* 阳; *niu xi* 牛膝, assisted by *chuan lian zi* 川楝子, is largely used to bring Blood downward; *mai ya* 麦芽 and *yin chen* 茵陈 sooth the Liver and relieve depressed emotion; *gan cao* 甘草 harmonizes all the above herbs.

Table 2.1 summarises the syndrome differentiation, treatment principles and key herbal formulas used in CHM for post-stroke shoulder pain.

Table 2.1 Summary of Syndrome Differentiation, Treatment Principles and Key Herbal Formulas

Syndrome	Treatment Principle	Key Formula
Wind-fire uprising	Calming the Liver and suppressing *yang* 阳, and clearing heat to eliminate Wind	Modified *Tian ma gou teng yin* 天麻钩藤饮加减
Wind-phlegm obstructing the collaterals	Eliminating Wind and reducing phlegm, activating Blood and unblocking collaterals	Modified *Hua tan tong luo tang* 化痰通络汤加减
Phlegm heat and excess in the *fu* 腑 organ	Reducing phlegm and clearing the *fu* 腑 organ.	Modified *Xing lou cheng qi tang* 星蒌承气汤加减
Qi 气 deficiency with Blood stasis	Tonifying *qi* 气 and activating Blood	Modified *Bu yang huan wu tang* 补阳还五汤加减
Yin 阴 deficiency with stirring Wind	Tonifying *yin* 阴 and suppressing *yang* 阳, calming the Liver and eliminating Wind	Modified *Zhen gan xi feng tang* 镇肝熄风汤加减

Topical Chinese Herbal Medicine Bath/Steam Therapy

CHM formula *Fu fang tong luo ye* 复方通络液 can be used for CHM bath/steam therapies. The main ingredients of *Fu fang tong luo ye* 复方通络液 are *hong hua* 红花, *chuan wu* 川乌, *cao wu* 草乌, *dang gui* 当归, *chuang xiong* 川芎 and *sang zhi* 桑枝. These herbs are mixed and boiled with water until 1,000–2,000 ml liquid remains. Use the warm CHM decoction to steam the affected limb, and later when the decoction is cooler, use it to wash or fomentate the affected limb.[2-4]

Acupuncture Therapies and Other Chinese Medicine Therapies

Body acupuncture: Select acupuncture points on *yangming* 阳明 meridians, in combination with points on *taiyang* 太阳 and *shaoyang* 少阳 meridians.

Selected points: LI15 *Jianyu* 肩髃, TE14 *Jianliao* 肩髎, SI9 *Jianzhen* 肩贞, (EX) *Jianqian* 肩前, *Ashi* points 阿是穴, TE2 *Yemen* 液门, TE4 *Yangchi* 阳池, SI4 *Wangu* 腕骨.[2]

Needling manipulation: Tonifying method or even method is often used; moxibustion is applicable.

Abdominal acupuncture points selection: CV12 *Zhongwan* 中脘, KI17 *Shangqu* 商曲 on the unaffected side, ST24 *Huaroumen* 滑肉门, etc. on the affected side.

Tuina 推拿 Therapy

Selected points: LI4 *Hegu* 合谷, LI11 *Quchi* 曲池, ST12 *Quepen* 缺盆, LI15 *Jianyu* 肩髃, SI9 *Jianzhen* 肩贞, GB21 *Jianjing* 肩井, SI11 *Tianzong* 天宗.

Manipulations: One-finger pushing, thumb pressing and/or flexed-finger pressing, pressing, grasping, pulling, traction and counter-traction, rocking, shaking and twisting.[3] Strong stimulation to spastic muscles should be avoided.

Other Management and Prevention Therapies

Patients with stroke in the acute stage need to be managed with proper positioning of the affected limb and regular changes of posture. When patients recover from unconsciousness or have stable vital signs, rehabilitation therapies should be applied as soon as possible. Meanwhile, proper positioning and supporting of the affected arm should always be applied. Patients with stroke should keep a good routine in their daily life, and regulate their diet and emotion. Since the aetiology of stroke often is initially vital *qi* 正气 deficiency in combination with unhealthy diet and extreme emotion, then the occurrence of unbalanced *yin* 阴 and *yang* 阳, and disordered *qi* 气 and Blood, therefore, it is important for middle-aged or aged stroke patients to do physical exercise regularly to keep healthy flow of *qi* 气 and Blood, to maintain pleasant mood and stable emotion, and to avoid fatty or heavy food and smoking or alcohol consumption.

References

1. 田德禄. (2002) 中医内科学. 北京: 人民卫生出版社.
2. 中国中医科学院. (2011) 中医循证临床实践指南 — 中医内科. 北京: 中国中医药出版社.
3. 中华中医药学会. (2008) 中医内科常见病诊疗指南·西医疾病部分. 北京: 中国中医药出版社.
4. 中华中医药学会. (2008) 中医内科常见病诊疗指南·中医疾病部分. 北京: 中国中医药出版社.
5. 彭怀仁. (1994) 中医方剂大辞典.北京: 人民卫生出版社.

3

Classical Chinese Medicine Literature

OVERVIEW

Classical Chinese medicine literature provides a rich source of information for prevention and management of disease. There may be some treatments used in contemporary practice that date back to classical literature, including current treatments for post-stroke complications. This chapter describes the findings of a systematic search of the *Zhong Hua Yi Dian* 中华医典, based on a selection of search terms identified from classical dictionaries and texts. Over 1,100 citations were analysed to identify the common formula, herbs and acupuncture points used to treat symptoms possibly, or likely to, correspond to post-stroke shoulder complications.

Introduction

Chinese medicine (CM) therapies have been practised for thousands of years. For example, acupuncture is commonly thought to originate in ancient China 2,500 years ago during the late Spring and Autumn period (770–476 BC) or early Warring States (474–221 BC) period,[1,2] and the book *Shen Nong Ben Cao Jing (Shennong's Materia Medica)* 神农本草经 is generally believed to be the oldest surviving book on materia medica presenting the earliest practice of Chinese herbal medicine (CHM) in the Western Han dynasty (206 BC–24 AD).[3,4]

During the thousands of years of CM clinical practice, a large amount of literature has accumulated which recorded descriptions of many diseases with symptoms similar to stroke and post-stroke complications. In order to explore the evidence of CM therapies for the management of stroke or its complications in history, it is important to systematically analyse the descriptions likely referring to these conditions in classical CM literature and discuss how they were conceptualised and managed over time. In order to systematically summarise such information from the vast classical CM literature, the digitalised collections *Zhong Hua Yi Dian* (ZHYD) 中华医典 CD-ROM — a collection of more than 1,000 medical books of the classical CM literature, was accessed. This collection is the largest currently available and is representative of other large collections of the classical and pre-modern CM literature.[3–5]

Clinically, stroke is characterised by a group of symptoms including:

- Muscular: Paralysis with weak muscles, problems with coordination, stiff muscle or paralysis of one side of the body;
- Whole body: Balance disorder, fatigue, light-headedness or vertigo;
- Visual: Blurred vision, double vision, sudden visual loss or temporary loss of vision in one eye;
- Speech: Difficulty speaking, slurred speech or speech loss;
- Sensory: Pins and needles or reduced sensation of touch;
- Facial: Muscle weakness or numbness;
- Limbs: Numbness or weakness;
- Also common: Difficulty swallowing, headache, inability to understand, limping or mental confusion.

Since stroke symptoms involve different parts of the body and may develop very fast, it was believed in the ancient CM concepts that this disease was corresponding to the features of Wind. Therefore, it was named *zhong feng* 中风 in Chinese language, which refers to 'a sudden Wind attack.'

The earliest record of 'Wind attack' dates back to the Spring and Autumn period and Warring States period (722–221 BC) in the book *Huang Di Nei Jing* 黄帝内经. However, symptoms of 'Wind attack' recorded in this book were more likely referring to the invasion of external pathogens rather than cerebrovascular accident. Nevertheless, the term *zhong feng* 中风 (Wind attack) did not always refer to the condition of stroke in history. On the other hand, there are some other terms which may not include the word *feng* 风 (Wind) but do, in fact, refer to this disease.

It has been pointed out that, since the era of *Huang Di Nei Jing* 黄帝内经 until the Qing dynasty (before 1911), there have been more than 30 terms used in different books referring to the condition of stroke. These terms include *pian ku* 偏枯, *pian feng* 偏风, *tan huan* 瘫缓, *zuo tan* 左瘫, *you huan* 右痪, *wei tui feng* 猥腿风, *da jue* 大厥, *jian jue* 煎厥, *bo jue* 薄厥, *pu ji* 仆击, *cu zhong* 卒中, *zhong feng* 中风, *fei feng* 肺风, *xin feng* 心风, *gan feng* 肝风, *pi feng* 脾风, *shen feng* 肾风, *fei zhong feng* 肺中风, *xin zhong feng* 心中风, *gan zhong feng* 肝中风, *pi zhong feng* 脾中风, *shen zhong feng* 肾中风, *nao feng* 脑风, *mu feng* 目风, *shou feng* 首风, *nei feng* 内风, *fei feng* 痱风, *feng qi* 风气, *wu fei* 瘖痱, *bao wu* 暴瘖, *feng yi* 风懿, *feng bi* 风痹, *wei feng* 微风, *lou feng* 漏风 and *lao feng* 劳风.[6] Therefore, to identify the treatments for stroke from CM classical literature requires clarification on the terminology used in the description.

Search Terms

Search terms were identified through a systematic screening process. Considering that post-stroke shoulder complications may not have been specifically discussed in history, we decided to search classical literature from an angle of overall stroke and post-stroke motor functional impairment.

Five CM books or clinical guidelines[7–11] and 20 journal articles or theses[12–31] on relevant topics were examined to identify potential search terms. A total of 61 terms were extracted and used in trial searches in the ZHYD. Through discussion of the preliminary results with clinical experts, 12 search terms were finally selected as most relevant to stroke. These were *zhong feng* 中风, *zhong jing* 中经, *zhong zang* 中脏, *bo jue* 薄厥, *cu zhong* (1) 猝中, *cu zhong* (2) 卒中, *feng fei* 风痱, *pian feng* 偏风, *pian ku* 偏枯, *tan huan* 瘫痪, *ban shen bu sui* (1) 半身不遂 and *ban shen bu sui* (2) 半身不随 (Table 3.1).

Table 3.1 Terms Used to Identify Classical Literature Citations

Search Terms in Pinyin	Search Terms in Chinese	English Translation
Zhong feng	中风	Sudden Wind attack
Zhong jing	中经	Hemiplegia-type dysfunction post-Wind attack
Zhong zang	中脏	Visceral stroke
Bo jue	薄厥	Flopping syncope
Cu zhong (1)	猝中	Sudden Wind attack
Cu zhong (2)	卒中	Sudden Wind attack
Feng fei	风痱	Sudden Wind attack
Pian feng	偏风	Hemiplegia-type Wind attack
Pian ku	偏枯	Hemiplegia-type dysfunction
Tan huan	瘫痪	Paralysis
Ban shen bu sui (1)	半身不遂	Hemiplegia
Ban shen bu sui (2)	半身不随	Hemiplegia

Procedures for Search, Data Coding and Data Analysis

Each term was entered into the ZHYD search fields and the search results were downloaded into spreadsheets (Fig. 3.1). The number of hits identified by each search term was calculated by summing the results of the searches.

Duplicate results caused by different search terms were removed. Codes were then allocated for types of citations, books and the dynasties in which they were written according to the procedures described in May *et al.*, 2014.[3]

A 'citation' was defined as a distinct passage of text referring to one or more of the search terms. All relevant citations were reviewed to identify the best descriptions of post-stroke motor functional impairment and its aetiology or pathogenesis.

Citations were excluded from further analyses if they were:

- Not related to stroke;
- Of paediatric diseases;

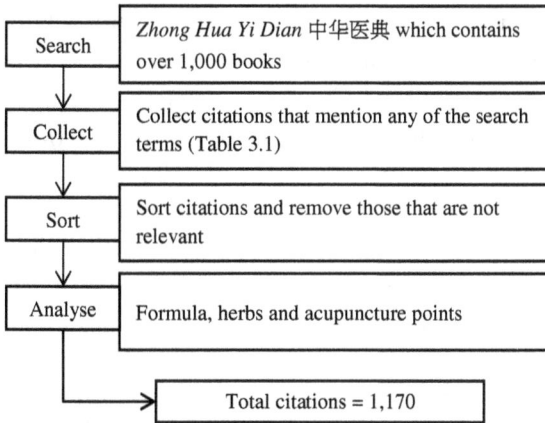

Fig. 3.1   Classical literature citations.

- Related to stroke but not about motor functional impairment;
- Related to post-stroke motor functional impairment but with a focus on the lower limb only;
- Not containing information of treatment.

Following exclusion, the final dataset was limited to the citations potentially referring to 'possibly related to post-stroke shoulder complications,' with description of CM treatments (CHM, acupuncture and related therapies, or other CM therapies). Included citations were grouped according to the CM intervention for further analysis. When a citation referred to multiple treatments, each treatment was considered as a separate citation for calculation of formulae, herbs, or acupuncture points. Citations which were pharmacopeia-type entries were reviewed for eligibility. Pharmacopeia entries which mentioned the name of the condition but did not include a detailed description of the condition, or information about treatment, were excluded from further analysis. Pharmacopeia entries which included a description of the condition, with or without reference to other herbs, were included.

Further, an additional screening process was performed to identify citations considered to be specifically related to post-stroke shoulder complications. Citations that mentioned shoulder or arm pain/dysfunction were selected to be the most 'likely related to post-stroke shoulder complications.' These citations were analysed following the same approach. Examples of such description are given:

Numbness and pain of the shoulder and arm (*jian bo ma mu* 肩膊麻痛), deep pain of the arm (*bi tong lian ji jin gu* 臂痛连及筋骨), shoulder and arm pain (*jian bi tong* 肩臂痛), arm pain (*bi teng tong* 臂疼痛), weakness of arm (*bi wu li* 臂无力), and difficulty in lifting arm to reach the head (*shou bu neng ji tou* 手不能及头).

At the end, all data were presented for the frequencies of identified formulae, herbs and acupuncture points within two levels: (1) citations which were possibly related to post-stroke shoulder complications and (2) citations which were likely related to post-stroke shoulder complications.

Search Results

A total of 27,460 instants (hits) were obtained using the 12 search terms; results are shown in Table 3.2. The search term which produced the highest number of hits was *zhong feng* 中风 (19,150 hits,

Table 3.2 Hit Frequency by Search Term

Pinyin	Chinese Characters	Hit Frequency (*n*, %)
Zhong feng	中风	19,150 (69.7)
Tan huan	瘫痪	1,532 (5.6)
Pian ku	偏枯	1,521 (5.5)
Ban shen bu sui (1)	半身不遂	1,380 (5.0)
Cu zhong (2)	卒中	1,261 (4.6)
Pian feng	偏风	907 (3.3)
Zhong zang	中脏	611 (2.2)
Zhong jing	中经	435 (1.6)
Bo jue	薄厥	208 (0.8)
Cu zhong (1)	猝中	206 (0.8)
Feng fei	风痱	204 (0.7)
Ban shen bu sui (2)	半身不随	45 (0.2)
Total		**27,460**

69.7%). All other search terms were identified in less than 6% of all hits (Table 3.2).

Citations Included for Analyses

After removal of duplicates and exclusions, a total of 1,170 citations were included as 'possibly related to post-stroke shoulder complications.' A total of 1,010 citations focused on CHM including CHM formula treatments, and 160 citations described some acupuncture-related therapies. Forty-eight citations reported clinical case reports.

Among all these included citations, 21 citations were further judged as 'likely related to post-stroke shoulder complications' since they specified symptoms of shoulder or upper limb. Of these, ten citations introduced CHM therapies and 11 citations focused on acupuncture therapies.

Definitions of the Condition and Aetiology

In addition to the citations containing treatments of CHM or acupuncture-related therapies, our search found around 1,000 citations describing the definition or aetiology of this condition without a treatment attached.

In ancient times, stroke (*zhong feng* 中风) was typically defined by symptoms. Examples are given below:

1. A person suddenly fell and the body became stiff, may present the symptoms of hemiplegia, bilateral limb paralysis or unconsciousness. This person may, or may not, die. It is called *zhong feng* 中风 (*Yi Jing Su Hui Ji* 医经溯洄集•中风辨, c 1368).
2. *Zhong feng* 中风 presents as a sudden fall, unconsciousness, large amount of sputum accumulated in the throat with snoring sound. The patient may present facial paralysis, bilateral limb paralysis or hemiplegia, mouth closed with lockjaw, stiff tongue and aphasia (*Yi Bian* 医碥•中风, c. 1751).
3. *Zhong feng* 中风 is a common name of the disease which presents as a sudden falling, facial paralysis, hemiplegia, stiff tongue with

aphasia, open mouth which cannot close. However, symptoms may vary from person to person; since it often presents as sudden falling, it used to be called *ji pu* 击仆 or *cu zhong* 卒中 because it is similar to Wind attack. For the symptoms of facial paralysis and hemiplegia, it used to be called *pian ku* 偏枯 or *zuo tan you huan* 左瘫右痪 (*Ji Yang Gang Mu* 济阳纲目•论风分在腑在脏在经浅深之异, c. 1626).

Other than the description of disease definition, there are some citations that discuss the aetiology of *zhong feng* 中风. The causality of this condition could be categorised as external pathogen, being overweight, and internal factors including internal Heat, deficiency and phlegm. Examples are listed below:

1. External pathogen with *qi* deficiency 气虚外邪:
   Pian ku 偏枯 is caused by deficiency of one side of the body. When there is deficiency of the defending *qi* 气, an external pathogen will attack this side of the body and cause disease (*Ling Shu* 灵枢•刺节真邪).
2. Being overweight/obesity素体肥胖:
   Pian ku 偏枯, and some other conditions, could be caused by being overweight/obese, it is also considered as disease caused by long-term intake of fatty food (*Su Wen* 素问•通评虚实论).
3. Internal factors:
   - Internal Heat 内热:
     Due to lack of resting, there is an internal Heart Fire growing. If such Heat is out of control, there will be *yin* deficiency and excess *yang*. The Heat will cause *qi* 气 being stagnated and therefore *shen* 神 becoming unclear, leading to sudden falling and unconsciousness (*He Jian Liu Shu* 河间六书•素问玄机原病式, c. 1601).
   - Internal deficiency 内虚:
     A condition named *fei feng* 非风, also commonly called *zhong feng* 中风. Symptoms include sudden falling, often accompanied by unconsciousness. This is caused by long-term internal deficiency rather than external Wind-cold invasion (*Jing Yue Quan Shu* 景岳全书•非风, c. 1624).

Zhong feng 中风 is not caused by external pathogen. In fact, it is caused by internal factors. In a person who is over 40 years old, his *qi* 气 starts to get weaker and weaker; if he also gets accumulated emotions, it will further damage the *qi* 气. Hence people in this age group commonly suffer from the condition of *zhong feng* 中风 but younger people are less likely to get it. In particular, people who are overweight are more likely to get this disease because the excess weight will further damage their *qi* 气 (*Yi Xue Fa Ming* 医学发明·中风有三, c. 1315).

- Internal Phlegm 痰蕴:

  People who live in the south-east may suffer from a type of 'Wind' disease. In fact, it is not real external Wind invasion. The real reason is middle-*jiao* 焦 Dampness causing Phlegm, Heat generated from the Phlegm, therefore internal Wind occurred (*Dan Xi Xin Fa* 丹溪心法·论中风).

  Most of the hemiplegia cases were caused by Phlegm. When the left side of the body is paralysed, it is due to dead Blood or insufficient Blood (*Dan Xi Xin Fa* 丹溪心法·论中风, c. 1481).

- Internal Wind 内风:

  For a person who has Blood and Essenes deficiency, water is not sufficient to nourish wood, hence Liver *yang* 阳 uprising causes internal Wind (*Lin Zheng Zhi Nan* 临证指南·中风, c. 1746).

  Doctor Hua recorded: Doctor Ye created the name of internal Wind 内风. It is due to unstable *yang qi* 阳气 of the body. Liver is known as both the wood organ and the wind organ, if the water is insufficient, the wood will not be nourished. Therefore, the Liver *yang* 阳 will raise and cause internal Wind. In this case, the treatment should consider nourishing *yin* 阴 and eliminating Wind (*Lin Zheng Zhi Nan Yi An* 临证指南医案·中风, c. 1746).

Chinese Herbal Medicine

A total of 1,010 included citations introduced CHM treatment. They were found in 235 books. The books with the largest number of citations are *Pu Ji Fang* 普济方 (*n* = 99), *Sheng Ji Zong Lu* 圣济总录

(*n* = 91), *Tai Ping Sheng Hui Fang* 太平圣惠方 (*n* = 74), *Ji Yang Gang Mu* 济阳纲目 (*n* = 41), *Qi Xiao Liang Fang* 奇效良方 (*n* = 28), *Gu Jin Yi Tong Da Quan* 古今医统大全 (*n* = 20), *Wai Tai Mi Yao* 外台秘要 (*n* = 20), *Tai Ping Hui Min He Ji Ju Fang* 太平惠民和剂局方 (*n* = 16), *Bei Ji Qian Jin Yao Fang* 备急千金要方 (*n* = 15) and *Yi Xue Gang Mu* 医学纲目 (*n* = 14).

Frequency of Treatment Citations by Dynasty

The majority of CHM treatment citations were identified in books from the Ming dynasty (c. 1369–1644) and Qing dynasty (c. 1645–1911), with almost two-thirds (64.5%) coming from this period (Table 3.3). Two citations were from books without known publishing years, and two citations were from a CHM book published in Japan (c. 1780) (see Table 3.3).

The earliest treatment citations were from *Hua Tuo Shen Fang* 华佗神方 (Han dynasty), with all three treatment citations coming from the same passage of text. These three treatments were identified by the search terms *zhong feng* 中风. The most recent citations were from the book named *Zhong Feng Jiao Quan* 中风斠诠 (c. 1917) and were identified by three search terms: *zhong feng* 中风, *ban shen bu sui* 半身不遂 and *pian feng* 偏风.

Table 3.3   Dynastic Distribution of Chinese Herbal Medicine Treatment Citations

Dynasty	No. of Treatment Citations
Before Tang dynasty (before 618)	4
Tang and Five dynasties (618–960)	45
Song and Jin dynasties (961–1271)	246
Yuan dynasty (1272–1368)	38
Ming dynasty (1369–1644)	396
Qing dynasty (1645–1911)	255
Ming Guo/Republic of China (1912–1949)	22
Others	2 unknown, 2 Japan*
Total	**1,010**

*Chinese medicine books published in Japan

The CHM treatments described in all included citations were analysed for frequency. If ingredients were not specified in the included citation, the book where the citation was found was searched to identify other instances of the same formula which listed the ingredients. If identified, these ingredients were used for analysis.

Treatment with Chinese Herbal Medicine

Citations that included interventions using Chinese herbal formulas were identified and categorised into those that were related to 'possible post-stroke shoulder complications' since they were used to treat one of the search terms and there were no reasons to exclude them as unlikely to have been associated with post-stroke motor function impairment. A subset of these citations, which mentioned shoulder or arm pain/dysfunction, was considered to be more likely to have referred to post-stroke shoulder complications.

Most Frequent Formulas in 'Possible Post-stroke Shoulder Complications' Citations

Of the 1,010 included CHM citations, 111 formulas contained unnamed combinations of herbs. A total of 474 named formulas were identified, with 158 formulas being described in multiple citations. The most frequently seen formulas are listed in Table 3.4. The herb ingredient list from the earliest citation is presented, as it is likely that earlier formulas were representative of subsequent formulas.

All these formulas were for oral ingestion. None of them are recommended in current key textbooks and clinical practice guidelines (see Chapter 2). This may be caused by, firstly, the different understanding of aetiology of stroke. As abovementioned, stroke was initially defined as external Wind attack, and later Kidney deficiency and Phlegm also played an important role in the aetiology. Secondly, citations which were considered to be treating stroke in general were all included in this level of analysis, thus these formulas seem not particularly focused on motor dysfunction.

Table 3.4   Most Frequent Formulas in 'Possible Post-stroke Shoulder Complications' Citations

Formula Name	Herb Ingredients	Number of Citations (*n*)
Da qin jiu tang 大秦艽汤	*Qin jiao* 秦艽, *gan cao* 甘草, *chuan xiong* 川芎, *dang gui* 当归, *bai shao* 白芍, *xi xin* 细辛, *qiang huo* 羌活, *fang feng* 防风, *huang qin* 黄芩, *shi gao* 石膏, *bai zhi* 白芷, *bai zhu* 白术, *shu di huang* 熟地黄, *fu ling* 茯苓 and *du huo* 独活 (*Su Wen Bing Ji Qi Yi Bao Ming Ji* 素问病机气宜保命集 c. 1108)	25
Modified *Si wu tang* 四物汤 加减	*Dang gui* 当归, *chuan xiong* 川芎, *bai shao* 白芍, *shu di huang* 熟地黄, *tao ren* 桃仁, *hong hua* 红花, *zhu li* 竹沥, *chen pi* 陈皮, *ban xia* 半夏, *fu ling* 茯苓, *gan cao* 甘草, *ji geng* 桔梗, *sheng jiang* 生姜 and *da zao* 大枣 (*Ren Shu Bian Lan* 仁术便览 c. 1585)	22
Xiao xu ming tang 小续命汤	*Ma huang* 麻黄, *rou gui* 肉桂, *gan cao* 甘草, *ren shen* 人参, *bai shao* 白芍, *chuan xiong* 川芎, *huang qin* 黄芩, *fang feng* 防风, *dang dui* 当归, *shi gao* 石膏, *bai zhu* 白术, *sheng jiang* 生姜, *fu zi* 附子 and *xing ren* 杏仁 (*Ren Zhai Zhi Zhi Fang Lun* 仁斋直指方论 c. 1264)	16
Xu ming tang 续命汤	*Ma huang* 麻黄, *gui zhi* 桂枝, *ren shen* 人参, *dang gui* 当归, *chuan xiong* 川芎, *shi gao* 石膏, *xing ren* 杏仁, *sheng jiang* 生姜 and *gan cao* 甘草 (*Jin Gui Yao Lue* 金匮要略 c. 205)	10
Modified *Liu jun zi tang* 六君子汤加减	*Ren shen* 人参, *bai zhu* 白术, *fu ling* 茯苓, *gan cao* 甘草, *chen pi* 陈皮 and *ban xia* 半夏, etc. (*Chi Shui Xuan Zhu* 赤水玄珠 c. 1584)	9
San huang tang 三黄汤	*Ma huang* 麻黄, *huang qi* 黄芪, *huang qin* 黄芩, *du huo* 独活 and *xi xin* 细辛 (*Sheng Ji Zong Lu* 圣济总录 c. 1117)	8

(Continued)

Table 3.4 (*Continued*)

Formula Name	Herb Ingredients	Number of Citations (n)
Wu yao shun qi san 乌药顺气散	*Wu yao* 乌药, *chen pi* 陈皮, *ma huang* 麻黄, *jiang can* 僵蚕, *chuan xiong* 川芎, *zhi shi* 枳实, *gan cao* 甘草, *jie geng* 桔梗, *bai zhi* 白芷, *sheng jiang* 生姜 and *da zao* 大枣 (*Qi Xiao Liang Fang* 奇效良方 c. 1470)	8
Di huang yin zi 地黄饮子	*Sheng di huang* 生地黄, *shu di huang* 熟地黄, *shi chang pu* 石菖蒲, *ba ji tian* 巴戟天, *fu zi* 附子, *rou gui* 肉桂, *shi hu* 石斛, *fu ling* 茯苓, *yuan zhi* 远志, *mai men dong* 麦门冬, *wu wei zi* 五味子, *bo he* 薄荷 and *shan zhu yu* 山茱萸 (*Cheng Fang Qie Yong* 成方切用 c. 1761)	8
Tian ma wan 天麻丸	1. *Tian ma* 天麻, *di yu* 地榆, *mo yao* 没药, *xuan shen* 玄参, *fu zi* 附子, *she xiang* 麝香, *feng mi* 蜂蜜, *jiu* 酒 2. *Tian ma* 天麻, *xuan shen* 玄参, *fang feng* 防风, *di yu* 地榆, *bo he* 薄荷, *fu zi* 附子, *niu xi* 牛膝, *zao jiao* 皂荚, *niu huang* 牛黄, *long nao* 龙脑, *jiu* 酒, *feng mi* 蜂蜜 and *fu ping* 浮萍 (*Sheng Ji Zong Lu* 圣济总录 c. 1117)	8
Zi shou jie yu tang 资寿解语汤	*Ling yang jiao* 羚羊角, *shi chang pu* 石菖蒲, *fang feng* 防风, *tian ma* 天麻, *qiang huo* 羌活, *gan cao* 甘草, *rou gui* 肉桂, *fu zi* 附子, *suan zao ren* 酸枣仁, *ban xia* 半夏, *xing ren* 杏仁, *zhi shi* 枳实 and *zhu li* 竹沥 (*Yi Fang Ji Yi* 医方集宜 c. 1644)	8

Note: 1. Formula ingredients are based on the earliest book within the group of included citations. 2. Formulas with the same name can vary in their ingredients and the same combination of ingredients may have different names. In this data, formulas with the same name that have variations in a few ingredients are grouped together, while those with large variations in ingredients are separated. Also, formulas with the same ingredients but different names have been grouped together. 3. The use of some herbs/ingredients may be restricted in some countries. For example, herbs such as *fu zi* 附子, *wu tou* 乌头 and *xi xin* 细辛 can be toxic, and some may be restricted under the Convention on International Trade in Endangered Species of Wild Fauna and Flora (CITES; e.g. *she xiang* 麝香). Readers are advised to comply with relevant regulations.

However, although these formulas are not consistent with those recommended in key textbooks and clinical practice guidelines, they may have some similarity in terms of the key herbs. Therefore, examining the actual herb ingredients is more meaningful.

Most Frequent Herbs in 'Possible Post-stroke Shoulder Complications' Citations

In the 1,010 included citations which described treatment with CHM, 415 different ingredients were included. It is noted that *jiu* 酒 was one of the most frequently used ingredients which was used in preparations to process the herbs. Also, *jiu* 酒 has the function of warming and smoothing meridians, which could be beneficial for treating post-stroke functional impairment. A selection of the most frequently used herbs are described in Table 3.5.

The most frequently used herb was *dang gui* 当归, used in 416 citations. *Dang gui* 当归 is commonly used as a Blood-moving herb to remove Blood stasis. *Fang feng* 防风 was also one of the most frequent herbs, since it was believed that stroke was caused by a sudden Wind attack; the use of *fang feng* 防风 was for the purpose of eliminating Wind. The third frequently used herb was *gan cao* 甘草; this is not surprising since *gan cao* 甘草 is frequently used to harmonise all ingredients in a formula.

It is noted that among these 20 herbs, there are some herbs that have the function of nourishing Blood and removing Blood stasis, e.g. *dang gui* 当归, *chuan xiong* 川芎, *di huang* 地黄 and *niu xi* 牛膝; some herbs could tonify *qi, yang* or Spleen, e.g. *fu zi* 附子, *wu tou* 乌头, *rou gui* 肉桂, *ren shen* 人参, *bai zhu* 白术, *fu ling* 茯苓 and ginger 生姜; some herbs may eliminate Wind, e.g. *fang feng* 防风, *qiang huo* 羌活, *ma huang* 麻黄, *xi xin* 细辛 and *qin jiu* 秦艽; and some herbs could work for opening up meridians, e.g. *tian ma* 天麻.

The inclusion of *fu zi* 附子, *wu tou* 乌头 and *xi xin* 细辛 is also noteworthy. These herbs are restricted in some countries due to their toxicity, and they are not recommended in current clinical guidelines as the treatment for post-stroke motor dysfunction. It is believed that the use of *fu zi* 附子 and *wu tou* 乌头 was for the purpose of

Table 3.5   Most Frequent Herbs in 'Possible Post-stroke Shoulder Complications' Citations

Herb Name	Scientific Name	No. of Citations (*n*)
Dang gui 当归	*Angelica sinensis* (Oliv.) Diels	416
Fang feng 防风	*Saposhnikovia divaricata* (Turcz.) Schischk.	407
Gan cao 甘草	Glycyrrhizae Radix et Rhizoma	387
Jiang/ sheng jiang 生姜, 姜	*Zingiber officinale* (Willd.) Rosc. (fresh or dried rhizome)	371
Chuan xiong 川芎	*Ligusticum chuanxiong* Hort.	361
Fu zi 附子	*Aconitum carmichaeli* Debx.	333
Rou gui 肉桂, 肉桂枝, 官桂	*Cinnamomum cassia* Presl	291
Ren shen 人参	*Panax ginseng* C.A. Mey.	280
Ma huang 麻黄	Ephedrae Herba	272
Di huang (*shu di huang/ sheng di huang/dihuang*) 地黄 (熟地黄/生地黄/地黄)	*Rehmannia glutinosa* Libosch.	248 (168/68/12)
Bai zhu 白术	*Atractylodes macrocephala* Koidz.	240
Qiang huo 羌活	*Notopterygium incisum* Ting ex H. T. Chang	*233*
Fu ling 茯苓	*Poria cocos* (Schw.) Wolf	215
Jiu 酒	Alcohol	214
Du huo 独活	*Angelica pubescens* Maxim. f. *biserrata* Shan et Yuan	211
Bai shao 白芍	*Paeonia lactiflora* Pall.	202
Tian ma 天麻	*Gastrodia elata* Bl.	202
Wu tou 乌头, 川乌, 草乌	1. *Aconitum carmichaeli* Debx. 2. *Aconitum kusnezoffii* Reichb.	161
Xi xin 细辛	1. *Asarum heterotropoides* Fr. Schmidt var. *mandshuricum* (Maxim) Kitag. 2. *Asarum sieboldii* Miq. var. *seoulense* Nakai 3. *Asarum sieboldii* Miq.	149
Niu xi 牛膝	*Cyathula officinalis* Kuan	145

Note: The use of some herbs, such as *fu zi* 附子, *wu tou* 乌头 and *xi xin* 细辛 may be restricted in some countries. Readers are advised to comply with relevant regulations.

warming and assisting the removal of Dampness/Phlegm. While *xi xin* 细辛 is often used in formulas eliminating external Wind, this reflects the fact that external Wind was considered as the cause of stroke in history.

Most Frequent Formulas in 'Likely Post-stroke Shoulder Complications' Citations

The 'likely post-stroke shoulder complications' citations are defined as those treatments for post-stroke motor functional impairment with a particular focus on the shoulder or upper limb. In total, ten citations were judged applicable in this category based on our symptom coding. They were attained from nine books: *Sheng Ji Zong Lu* 圣济总录 (*n* = 2), *Wan Bing Hui Chun* 万病回春 (*n* = 1), *Qian Jin Yi Fang* 千金翼方 (*n* = 1), *Tai Yi Yuan Mi Cang Gao Dan Wan San Fang Ji* 太医院秘藏膏丹丸散方剂 (*n* = 1), *Tai Ping Hui Min He Ji Ju Fang* 太平惠民和剂局方 (*n* = 1), *Qi Xiao Liang Fang* 奇效良方 (*n* = 1), *Shou Shi Bao Yuan* 寿世保元 (*n* = 1), *Jiao Zhu Fu Ren Liang Fang* 校注妇人良方 (*n* = 1) and *Zheng Zhi Zhun Sheng — Lei Fang* 证治准绳·类方 (*n* = 1).

Nine formulas were found from these citations, with only one formula appearing twice (*Shi wei cuo san* 十味锉散). *Shi wei cuo san* 十味锉散 was shown in two citations from two books of the Ming dynasty (*Qi Xiao Liang Fang* 奇效良方 and *Zheng Zhi Zhun Sheng — Lei Fang* 证治准绳·类方, c. 1602). In both citations this formula was stated as treating Blood deficiency type *zhong feng* 中风, upper limb pain and difficult movement (治中风血弱, 臂痛连及筋骨, 举动艰难).

Other formulas found in this pool include *Wu yao shun qi san* 乌药顺气散, modified *Si wu tang* plus *Hong hua jian* 四物汤合红花煎加减, *Wu bi gao* 无比膏 (topical application), *Hai tong pi wan* 海桐皮丸, *Shen xiao huo luo dan* 神效活络丹, *Lu gong jiu* 鲁公酒, *Hei shen wan* 黑神丸 and *Di huang wan* 地黄丸. However, since these formulas have not been shown repeatedly; their use for treating post-stroke shoulder complications remains uncertain.

Most Frequent Herbs in 'Likely Post-stroke Shoulder Complications' Citations

By analysing the ingredients of these nine formulas, a total of 65 herbs were found. Fourteen ingredients were shown in at least two citations (see Table 3.6).

It is worth noting that, except for one herb (*shi hu* 石斛), all of the other 13 ingredients are also included as the most frequently used herbs of all CHM citations.

Table 3.6 Most Frequent Herbs in 'Likely Post-stroke Shoulder Complications' Citations

Herb Name	Scientific Name	No. of Citations (*n*)
Chuan xiong 川芎	*Ligusticum chuanxiong* Hort.	4
Di huang (*shu di huang/di huang*) 地黄 (熟地黄/地黄)	*Rehmannia glutinosa* Libosch.	4 (2/2)
Fu zi 附子	*Aconitum carmichaeli* Debx.	3
Jiang 生姜, 姜	*Zingiber officinale* (Willd.) Rosc. (fresh or dried rhizome)	3
Fang feng 防风	*Saposhnikovia divaricata* (Turcz.) Schischk.	3
Bai shao 白芍	*Paeonia lactiflora* Pall.	3
Shi hu 石斛	1. *Dendrobium nobile* Lindl. 2. *Dendrobium chysotoxum* Lindl. 3. *Dendrobium fimbriatum* Hook.	2
Niu xi 牛膝	*Cyathula officinalis* Kuan	2
Rou gui 肉桂, 肉桂枝, 官桂	*Cinnamomum cassia* Presl	2
Gan cao 甘草	Glycyrrhizae Radix et Rhizoma	2
Wu tou 乌头, 川乌, 草乌	1. *Aconitum carmichaeli* Debx. 2. *Aconitum kusnezoffii* Reichb.	2
Dang gui 当归	*Angelica sinensis* (Oliv.) Diels	2
Ma huang 麻黄	Ephedrae Herba	2
Jiu 酒	Alcohol	2

Note: The use of some herbs such as *fu zi* 附子 and *wu tou* 乌头 may be restricted in some countries. Readers are advised to comply with relevant regulations.

Representative Citations

Our search of ZHYD did not find any case report with clear description of post-stroke shoulder complications, suggesting that shoulder complications were not considered to require specific treatment in the past. The one which is close to shoulder-hand syndrome is the *Shi wei cuo san* 十味锉散 citation from *Qi Xiao Liang Fang* 奇效良方 (c. 1470).

There was one theory proposed by Zhu Danxi in his book *Dan Xi Xin Fa* (丹溪心法·中风, c. 1481) stating that if hemiplegia occurs on the left side of body, it is due to Blood stasis; while if it occurs on the right side of the body it should be due to Phlegm and Heat in combination with *qi* 气 deficiency. Therefore, the treatments for different side hemiplegia should also be different. This method had been repeatedly quoted by a number of books in the Ming dynasty.

Discussion of Chinese Herbal Medicine

In summary, a total of 1,010 citations introduced CHM formula treatments for post-stroke functional impairment, possibly including shoulder complications. Of these, ten citations contained particular shoulder or upper limb symptoms and therefore were selected as the most representative pool.

A total of 474 named CHM formulas containing 415 different ingredients were identified from all included CHM citations. One-hundred and fifty-eight formulas had been introduced by multiple citations with four formulas being used in more than ten citations: *Da qin jiu tang* 大秦艽汤, modified *Si wu tang* 四物汤加减, *Xiao xu ming tang* 小续命汤 and *Xu ming tang* 续命汤. The most frequently used herbs of these citations showed the function of nourishing Blood and removing Blood stasis; tonifying *qi* 气, Spleen or Kidney; reducing Phlegm; eliminating Wind; and opening up meridians. This reflected the main focuses of the aetiology of stroke in the historical understanding. Such treatment principles are similar to those currently being used, although the formulas are not recommended by clinical guidelines (see Chapter 2). In particular, the treatment purposes of tonifying *qi* 气, removing Blood stasis and opening up meridians are consistent with that of *Bu yang huan wu tang* 补阳还五汤, the key formula being recommended by clinical guidelines to treat post-stroke functional impairment.

Ten citations were further selected since they contained information on post-stroke motor functional impairment with a particular focus on shoulder or upper limb. Nine formulas were introduced by these citations, with *Shi wei cuo san* 十味锉散 being repeatedly used. The symptoms treated by this formula are similar to shoulder-hand syndrome. However, due to the small number of formulas and herbs, we cannot draw any clear conclusion on their use for post-stroke shoulder complications.

It has been noted that some herbs used in history are no longer in use in current clinical practice. For example, *she xiang* 麝香 is produced from endangered animals and is restricted under the provisions of the Convention on International Trade in Endangered Species of Wild Fauna and Flora (CITES). In addition, some herbs such as *fu zi* 附子, *wu tou* 乌头 and *xi xin* 细辛 may be restricted in some countries due to their toxicity. In fact, the toxicity of *fu zi* 附子 and *wu tou* 乌头 was not neglected in ancient China. The book *Dan Xi Xin Fa* 丹溪心法, written in 1347 AD, stated that adding a small amount of *fu zi* 附子 and *wu tou* 乌头 into the CHM formula was suitable for people of Dampness type, because these two herbs could assist other tonifying herbs to resolve the Dampness and Phlegm. It was also pointed out that, in order to reduce the toxicity of *fu zi* 附子 and *wu tou* 乌头, special herbal processing approaches were needed.

Acupuncture and Related Therapies

A total of 160 citations stated acupuncture or moxibustion treatments for symptoms 'possibly related to post-stroke shoulder complications'. They were found in 33 books; the most cited ones are *Pu Ji Fang — Zhen Jiu* 普济方•针灸 (*n* = 20), *Gu Jin Yi Tong Da Quan* 古今医统大全 (*n* = 15), *Lei Jing Tu Yi* 类经图翼 (*n* = 11), *Zhen Jiu Da*

Cheng 针灸大成 (*n* = 10), *Tai Ping Sheng Hui Fang* 太平圣惠方 (*n* = 9), *Zhen Jiu Ji Cheng* 针灸集成 (*n* = 9), *Zhen Jiu Ju Ying* 针灸聚英 (*n* = 8), *Sheng Ji Zong Lu* 圣济总录 (*n* = 7), *Mian Xue Tang Zhen Jiu Ji Cheng* 勉学堂针灸集成 (*n* = 6) and *Zhen Fang Liu Ji* 针方六集 (*n* = 6).

Frequency of Treatment Citations by Dynasty

Similar to the CHM citations, the majority of these citations were identified in books from the Ming dynasty (c. 1369–1644) and Qing dynasty (c. 1645–1911). The earliest treatment citations were from *Huang Di Ming Tang Jiu Jing* 黄帝明堂灸经 (c. 1341) and the most recent citations were from the book *Jin Zhen Mi Zhuan* 金针秘传 (c. 1937). Five citations were from books without known publishing years, and one citation was from a Japanese acupuncture textbook published in the Qing dynasty (Table 3.7).

Treatment with Acupuncture-related Therapies

Of the 160 included acupuncture citations, 110 were from the angle of introducing the functions of acupuncture points. These citations stated that a particular acupuncture point could be used for treating

Table 3.7   Dynastic Distribution of Acupuncture Treatment Citations

Dynasty	No. of Treatment Citations
Before Tang dynasty (before 618)	0
Tang and Five dynasties (618–960)	6
Song and Jin dynasties (961–1271)	24
Yuan dynasty (1272–1368)	8
Ming dynasty (1369–1644)	79
Qing dynasty (1645–1911)	35
Ming Guo/Republic of China (1912–1949)	2
Others	5 unknown, 1 Japan*
Total	**160**

*Chinese medicine book published in Japan

certain clinical conditions or symptoms. Two citations recorded clinical case reports. The acupuncture points described in all these citations were analysed for frequency.

Frequently Used Acupuncture Points in 'Possible Post-stroke Shoulder Complications' Citations

A total of 96 acupuncture points were found in all included acupuncture citations. The top ones are presented in Table 3.8.

Table 3.8 Most Frequent Points in 'Possible Post-stroke Shoulder Complications' Citations

Acupuncture Points	No. of Citations (*n*)
LI11 *Quchi* 曲池	41
LI15 *Jianyu* 肩髃	32
GV20 *Baihui* 百会	23
LI10 *Shousanli* 手三里	22
GB31 *Fengshi* 风市	20
GB30 *Huantiao* 环跳	19
LU7 *Lieque* 列缺	18
GB39 *Xuanzhong* 悬钟	17
LI4 *Hegu* 合谷	15
GB34 *Yanglingquan* 阳陵泉	15
BL60 *Kunlun* 昆仑	12
CV24 *Chengjiang* 承浆	11
GB21 *Jianjing* 肩井	10
ST36 *Zusanli* 足三里	10
BL40 *Weizhong* 委中	7
GB3 *Shangguan* 上关	7
ST4 *Dicang* 地仓	6
KI6 *Zhaohai* 照海	6
GV16 *Fengfu* 风府	5
GB40 *Qiuxu* 丘墟	5
ST6 *Jiache* 颊车	5
BL15 *Xinshu* 心俞	5
GB2 *Tinghui* 听会	5
GB20 *Fengchi* 风池	5
GB38 *Yangfu* 阳辅	5

According to the locations and functions, these acupuncture points can be grouped as listed below:

Upper limb: LI11 *Quchi* 曲池, LI15 *Jianyu* 肩髃, LI10 *Shousanli* 手三里, LU7 *Lieque* 列缺, LI4 *Hegu* 合谷 and GB21 *Jianjing* 肩井.

Lower limb: GB31 *Fengshi* 风市, GB30 *Huantiao* 环跳, GB34 *Yanglingquan* 阳陵泉, BL60 *Kunlun* 昆仑, ST36 *Zusanli* 足三里, BL40 *Weizhong* 委中, GB39 *Xuanzhong* 悬钟, KI6 *Zhaohai* 照海, GB38 *Yangfu* 阳辅 and GB40 *Qiuxu* 丘墟.

Facial area: CV24 *Chengjiang* 承浆, GB3 *Shangguan* 上关, ST4 *Dicang* 地仓, GB2 *Tinghui* 听会 and ST6 *Jiache* 颊车.

To clear the mind and *shen* 神: GV20 *Baihui* 百会 and BL15 *Xinshu* 心俞.

To eliminate wind: GV16 *Fengfu* 风府 and GB20 *Fengchi* 风池.

However, since there are no specific criteria placed on the citations in this level, these acupuncture points are not considered limited to post-stroke shoulder complications. They are, in fact, the points used in general acupuncture treatment for stroke.

Most of these points were suggested to be used for both acupuncture and moxibustion, for example, 'using point LI9 *Shanglian* 上廉 for treatment, needling for 0.5 *cun* 寸 and apply five moxibustion on it; for the point LI10 *Shousanli* 手三里, needling for 0.2 *cun* 寸 and apply three moxibustion on it.'

There is one case report found which provided a detailed description of stroke-like symptoms. It is from a book published in 1937 (*Jin Zhen Mi Zhuan* 金针秘传). The symptom of slight hand/foot numbness may often be neglected; however, without proper treatment such symptoms may lead to severe stroke. Such a description is somehow similar to the concept of a transient ischaemic attack (TIA) or 'mini-stroke', which is a serious warning sign that a stroke may happen later (see below):

'When having numbness on the hand or foot, people usually do not pay much attention to it. However, they are not aware that this could be the beginning of wind diseases. If this is not treated in the early stage, it may develop into other conditions; some may be life-threatening including cerebrovascular accident and heart attack. According to Chinese medicine theory, they are under the category of *zhong feng* 中风' (*Jin Zhen Mi Zhuan* 金针秘传).

Frequently Used Acupuncture Points in 'Likely Post-stroke Shoulder Complications' Citations

By placing the criteria of 'shoulder or upper limb specific symptoms,' the included acupuncture citations pool was narrowed down to 11 citations. They were obtained from nine books including *Bian Que Shen Ying Zhen Jiu Yu Long Jing* 扁鹊神应针灸玉龙经 (*n* = 2), *Lei Jing Tu Yi* 类经图翼 (*n* = 2), *Pu Ji Fang — Zhen Jiu* 普济方•针灸 (*n* = 1), *Tai Ping Sheng Hui Fang* 太平圣惠方 (*n* = 1), *Wei Sheng Bao Jian* 卫生宝鉴 (*n* = 1), *Gu Jin Yi Tong Da Quan* 古今医统大全 (*n* = 1), *Zhen Jiu Wen Dui* 针灸问答 (*n* = 1), *Jiu Fa Mi Chuan* 灸法秘传 (*n* = 1) and *Zhen Fang Liu Ji* 针方六集 (*n* = 1).

A total of ten acupuncture points was found from these citations, with only three points being shown in multiple citations (Table 3.9). Other points which were only included in one citation for each were LU5 *Chize* 尺泽, LI10 *Shousanli* 手三里, LI4 *Hegu* 合谷, LU7 *Lieque* 列缺, SI4 *Wangu* 腕骨, SI3 *Houxi* 后溪 and GV20 *Baihui* 百会.

LI15 *Jianyu* 肩髃 is included in 54.5% citations (*n* = 6) indicating that it could be promising to use this point for post-stroke shoulder complications. For example, it could be used for moxibustion when treating or preventing post-stroke shoulder subluxation:

'Dr Wang said that if a person is feeling cold and painful in the shoulders, this should not be ignored. I have seen stroke patients

Table 3.9 Most Frequent Points in 'Likely Post-stroke Shoulder Complications' Citations

Acupuncture Points	No. of Citations (*n*)
LI15 Jianyu 肩髃	6
GB21 Jianjing 肩井	2
LI11 Quchi 曲池	2

presenting shoulder luxation resulting in the arm being out of the shoulder joint, such condition may not be cured. Therefore, when a person is feeling cold and painful in the shoulder, moxibustion on LI15 *Jianyu* 肩髃 should be applied to avoid the irreversible problem' (*Pu Ji Fang* 普济方•针灸•肩痹痛, c. 1410).

LI15 *Jianyu* 肩髃 can also be used for both acupuncture and moxibustion for the treatment of post-stroke shoulder pain and dysfunction:

'LI15 *Jianyu* 肩髃 is located at …This point can be used for needling for 0.6 *cun* 寸 and retain the needle for the duration of six breaths, then apply moxibustion on the point for three to 49 *zhuang* 壮. This can be the treatment of *zhong feng* 中风, hemiplegia, shoulder and arm pain and limited shoulder function' (*Lei Jing Tu Yi* 类经图翼•手阳明大肠经穴, c. 1624).

Discussion of Acupuncture

Our search of ZHYD found that the acupuncture treatment for *zhong feng* 中风 dates back to the Tang dynasty, and had been continually used until current clinical practice. It is found by our review that the earliest description of likely post-stroke shoulder subluxation treated with acupuncture is from the book published in the Song dynasty, *Tai Ping Sheng Hui Fang* 太平圣惠方 (c. 922).

There were a total of 160 citations identified as acupuncture treatment for post-stroke functional impairment possibly including shoulder complications. When the criteria were limited to 'shoulder or upper limb specific symptoms,' only 11 citations were included in the most representative pool.

A total of 96 acupuncture points was identified from all included citations. Similar to current clinical practice, the principle of selecting acupuncture points in the treatments for post-stroke functional impairment is firstly choosing the points in the diseased area, assisted by CM syndrome differentiation. By focusing the symptoms to be on shoulder and upper limb only, the promising acupuncture points were limited to three points located on the shoulder and upper limb: LI15 *Jianyu* 肩髃, GB21 *Jianjing* 肩井 and LI11 *Quchi* 曲池. Most of the points could be used for both acupuncture and moxibustion. It should be highlighted that LI15 *Jianyu* 肩髃 could be considered as the key acupuncture point for treating and preventing post-stroke shoulder complications.

Classical Literature in Perspective

In the history of CM, *zhong feng* 中风 was defined based on its symptoms. Different terms may refer to different stages or complications of stroke. The acute stage with unconsciousness could be named *pu ji* 仆击, *da jue* 大厥, *po jue* 薄厥; hemiplegia may be called *ban shen bu sui* 半身不遂, *pian ku* 偏枯, *pian feng* 偏风, *feng fei* 风痱; and aphasia was described using *yin fei* 喑痱. However, there has not been a specific disease name referring to post-stroke shoulder complications. Therefore, we screened all citations related to stroke and selected those that contained descriptions of shoulder/upper limb symptoms.

Zhong feng 中风 refers to 'a sudden Wind attack.' The concept of 'Wind' in stroke was initially external pathogen then developed to be internal factors. In *Huang Di Nei Jing* 黄帝内经, the causality of this disease was said to be external pathogen invasion together with *qi* 气 deficiency. Being overweight/obesity was noted as a potential risk factor of *pian ku* 偏枯 in *Huang Di Nei Jing* 黄帝内经. In the Han dynasty, *Zhang Zhongjing* 张仲景 proposed to classify *zhong feng* 中风 into *zhong jing* 中经, *zhong luo* 中络, *zhong zang* 中脏 and *zhong fu* 中腑 based on symptom severity. The causality of *zhong feng* 中风 started to be switched to internal factors in the Song dynasty, the deficiency of *zang fu* 脏腑 and *qi* 气, and Blood was emphasised to be the fundamental factors of Wind attack. The Jin and Yuan dynasties were the milestones in the history of stroke aetiology development. In these periods, physicians suggested that *zhong feng* 中风 was caused by internal factors rather than external pathogens. *Zhu Danxi* 朱丹溪 pointed out that *zhong feng* 中风 was the result of a combination of multiple internal pathogens including deficiency of *qi* 气 and Blood, Phlegm, Blood stasis and Heat. However, *Zhu Danxi* 朱丹溪 claimed that hemiplegia on different sides of the body was caused by different reasons; this is an incorrect theory. In the Ming dynasty, Liver *yang* 阳 upraising became the dominating aetiology of *zhong feng* 中风. In the Minguo period, along with the spread of western medicine, Chinese physician *Zhang Xichun* 张锡纯 adopted the two types of stroke (ischaemic, due to lack of blood flow; and haemorrhagic, due to bleeding) and put forward the name of *nao pin xue* 脑贫血 and *nao chong xue* 脑充血 (*Yi Xue Zhong Zhong Can Xi Lu* 医学衷中参西录, c. 1924).

With regard to CHM treatment, the formulas found in our classical literature review are not completely consistent with what are used in current clinical practice (see Table 3.4). This could be due to the following reasons: (1) some formulas were often used in the acute stage of stroke; however, in current practice, CHM does not play an important role in this stage; (2) formula names changed over time along with modification. For example, modified *Si wu tang* 四物汤加减 was a frequently used formula stated in classical literature, while *Bu yang huan wu tang* 补阳还五汤 is also a modified form of *Si wu tang* 四物汤; however, it was named in the Qing dynasty. Therefore, it was identified by our search but with low frequency; (3) in current clinical practice, formulas such as *Shen tong zhu yu tang* 身痛逐瘀汤, *Du huo ji sheng tang* 独活寄生汤 and *Huang qi wu wu gui zhi tang* 黄芪桂枝五物汤 are commonly used for post-stroke shoulder complications based on their effectiveness for pain relief. Since they were not recorded in classical literature in the management for stroke, they were not frequently shown in our classical literature search.

On the other hand, the frequently used herb ingredients were similar to what are in use currently (see Table 3.5). The function of those herbs included nourishing Blood and removing Blood stasis; tonifying *qi* 气, Spleen or Kidney; reducing Phlegm; eliminating Wind; and opening up meridians. Although some toxic herbs such as *wu tou* 乌头 and *fu zi* 附子 were frequently used, people did make efforts to detoxify these.

Acupuncture and moxibustion had been used in ancient China for the treatment of post-stroke functional impairment. Our search of ZHYD found that LI15 *Jianyu* 肩髃, GB21 *Jianjing* 肩井 and LI11 *Quchi* 曲池 are the acupuncture points used for likely post-stroke shoulder complications, with LI15 *Jianyu* 肩髃 being considered as the key acupuncture point.

Our review of classical literature did not identify *tuina* 推拿 therapy or other CM therapy for post-stroke shoulder complications. Except for using moxibustion on LI15 *Jianyu* 肩髃, other common management or prevention approaches, such as positioning or strapping, were not recorded in the classical literature.

References

1. Ma KW. (2000) Acupuncture: Its place in the history of Chinese medicine. *Acupunct Med* **18**(2): 88–99.

2. White A, Ernst E. (2004) A brief history of acupuncture. *Rheumatology* (Oxford) **43**(5): 662–663.

3. May BH, Lu Y, Lu C, *et al.* (2013) Systematic assessment of the representativeness of published collections of the traditional literature on Chinese medicine. *J Altern Complement Med* **19**(5): 403–409.

4. May BH, Lu C, Xue CC. (2012) Collections of traditional Chinese medical literature as resources for systematic searches. *J Altern Complement Med* **18**(12): 1101–1107.

5. Jia Hong Science and Technology Development Co. Ltd. (2014) *Zhong Hua Yi Dian* 中华医典 (ZHYD) [Encyclopaedia of Traditional Chinese Medicine, 5th ed], Electronic and Audio-Visual Publishing House, Changsha, Hunan.

6. 吴朋骉. (2005) 黄芪桂枝五物汤治疗中风的现代文献研究 [Thesis]. 北京中医药大学.

7. 周仲英. (2007) 中医内科学. 中国中医药出版社.

8. 张伯礼. (2012) 中医内科学. 人民卫生出版社.

9. 田德禄, 蔡淦. (2013) 中医内科学. 上海科学技术出版社.

10. 王永炎, 谢雁鸣. (2010) 实用中风病康复学. 人民卫生出版社.

11. 中国中医科学院. (2011) 中医循证临床实践指南:中医内科分册. 中国中医药出版社.

12. 高驰, 朱建平. (2014) '中风' 病名源流考. 中华中医药杂志 (05): 1298–1303.

13. 郜峦, 王键. (2009) 中风病病因病机的源流及发展. 中国中医急症 (08): 1279–1281.

14. 龚彪, 邹敏, 罗华丽. (2006) 从中风的诊断探讨中医的病名诊断. 陕西中医学院学报 (02): 11–12.

15. 黄伟贞. (2014) 西医脑出血与中医中风病病名诊断的对比研究. 现代中西医结合杂志 (07): 690–692.

16. 金栋. (2009) '卒中' 病名考. 世界中西医结合杂志 (03): 156–158.

17. 金栋. (2009) 古病名 '痱病' 探源. 世界中西医结合杂志 (05): 310–311.

18. 李红香. (2011) 基于中医文献的中风病研究 [Thesis]. 南京中医药大学.

19. 李红香, 戴慎. (2011) 中风病名探源. 辽宁中医药大学学报 (04): 158–159.

20. 李长君. (2007) 针灸治疗中风病的文献研究 [Thesis]. 黑龙江中医药大学.

21. 梁天坚. (2015) 叶天士痱中病名及证治简析. 江苏中医药 (08): 7–8.

22. 刘伍立, 欧阳建军, 黄博辉. (2006) 中医文献对中风病的阐述与述评. 针灸临床杂志 (10): 5–8+66.

23. 王春虎, 张运克. (2014) 中风病名新解. 中医临床研究 (31): 47–48.

24. 王建华. (1997) 真中风类中风源流概述. 河北中医 (04): 45–47.

25. 温春胜. (2013) 中风病中西医病名诊断的对比研究 [Thesis]. 广西医科大学.

26. 徐木林. (1996) 中风之古与今. 辽宁中医杂志 (06): 253–254.

27. 许玉皎. (2011) 中风病名分析及现代中风病诊断. 中医药导报 (05): 6–8.

28. 杨海涛, 张冬梅, 谢天. (2014) 中风病名溯源. 中国社区医师 (06): 10–11.

29. 张碧生. (2012) 中风源流考辩及其辨证论治规律 [Thesis]. 山东中医药大学.

30. 赵永辰. (2008) '中风' 病名探源及病机沿革. 中华中医药杂志 (04): 290–292.

31. 赵正孝. (2003) 中医中风病的诊治思想及源流研究 [Thesis]. 湖南中医学院.

4

Methods for Evaluating Clinical Evidence

OVERVIEW

This chapter describes the methods used to identify and evaluate a range of Chinese medicine interventions for post-stroke shoulder complications in clinical studies. Studies identified through a comprehensive search were assessed against eligibility criteria. A review of the methodological quality of the studies was undertaken using standardised methods. Results from the included studies were evaluated to provide an estimate of the effects of a range of Chinese medicine therapies.

Introduction

The use of Chinese medicine (CM) for post-stroke motor function has been well described in the CM contemporary literature and recorded in classical literature. It was also identified that various systematic reviews have been conducted to evaluate the efficacy and safety of CM treatments for post-stroke shoulder complications. These included five reviews of acupuncture related therapies (see Chapter 7), and two reviews of *tuina* 推拿 therapy (see Chapter 8).

This chapter describes the methods used to evaluate clinical studies, which are presented in subsequent chapters. Studies were evaluated following the methods of the Cochrane Handbook of Systematic Reviews.[1] Interventions have been categorised as follows:

- Chinese herbal medicine (CHM) (Chapter 5);
- Acupuncture and related therapies (Chapter 7);

Table 4.1   Chinese Medicine Interventions Included in Clinical Evidence Evaluation

Category	Intervention
Chinese herbal medicines	Oral, bath therapy, fomentation and external application
Acupuncture and related therapies	Acupuncture, electroacupuncture, scalp acupuncture, acupressure, floating acupuncture and moxibustion
Other Chinese medicine therapies	*Tuina* 推拿 therapy (Chinese massage) and cupping therapy
Combination of Chinese medicine therapies	Combination therapies are defined as two or more Chinese medicine interventions from different categories administered together, e.g. Chinese herbal medicines plus acupuncture or Chinese herbal medicines plus *tuina* 推拿 therapy

- Other CM therapies (Chapter 8);
- Combination CM therapies (Chapter 9).

References to clinical trials were obtained and assessed by an expert group. Randomised controlled trials (RCTs), non-randomised controlled clinical trials (CCTs) and non-controlled studies were evaluated in detail. Non-randomised controlled clinical trials were evaluated using the same approach as RCTs, and have been described separately. Evidence from non-controlled studies is more difficult to evaluate, therefore the approach was taken to describe the characteristics of the study, details of the intervention and any adverse events. References to included studies are indicated by a letter followed by a number. Studies of CHM are indicated by a 'H' e.g. H1, studies of acupuncture and related therapies are indicated by an 'A' e.g. A1, studies of other CM therapies are indicated by an 'O' e.g. O1, and studies of combinations of CM therapies (see Table 4.1) indicated by a 'C' e.g. C1.

Search Strategy

Evidence was searched in English- and Chinese-language databases and the methods followed the Cochrane Handbook of Systematic

Reviews.[1] English-language databases included PubMed, Excerpta Medica Database (Embase), Cumulative Index of Nursing and Allied Health Literature (CINAHL), Cochrane Central Register of Controlled Trials (CENTRAL) and Allied and Complementary Medicine Database (AMED). Chinese-language databases included China BioMedical Literature (CBM), China National Knowledge Infrastructure (CNKI), Chonqing VIP (CQVIP) and Wanfang. Databases were searched from inception to May 2015. No restrictions were applied. Search terms were mapped to controlled vocabulary (where applicable), in addition to being searched as keywords.

To conduct a comprehensive search of the literature, searches were run according to the study design (reviews, controlled trials and non-controlled studies). This was done for each of the three intervention types (CHM, acupuncture and related therapies, and other CM therapies) resulting in nine searches in each of the nine databases:

1. CHM reviews;
2. CHM controlled trials (randomised and non-randomised);
3. CHM non-controlled studies;
4. Acupuncture and related therapies — reviews;
5. Acupuncture and related therapies — controlled trials (randomised and non-randomised);
6. Acupuncture and related therapies — non-controlled studies;
7. Other CM therapies — reviews;
8. Other CM therapies — controlled trials (randomised and non-randomised);
9. Other CM therapies — non-controlled studies.

Studies of combination CM therapies were identified through the above searches. In addition to electronic databases, reference lists of systematic reviews and included studies were searched for additional publications. Clinical trial registries were searched to identify clinical trials which were ongoing or completed, and where required, trial investigators were contacted to obtain data. The searched trial registries included the Australian New Zealand Clinical Trial Registry (ANZCTR), the Chinese Clinical Trial Registry (ChiCTR), the European

Union Clinical Trials Register (EU-CTR) and the US National Institutes of Health register (ClinicalTrials.gov).

Inclusion Criteria

- Participants: Patients who developed post-stroke (ischaemic or haemorrhagic type) shoulder complications, including shoulder pain, subluxation and shoulder-hand syndrome; the stroke diagnosis was confirmed by computed tomography (CT) or magnetic resonance imaging (MRI) scan;
- Interventions: CHM, acupuncture and related therapies, or other CM therapies, alone or in combination with other CM therapies or with pharmacotherapy/routine rehabilitation (see Table 4.1 for details). Studies combining CM therapies with pharmacotherapy/ routine rehabilitation were required to use the same pharmacotherapy/routine rehabilitation in both the intervention and comparator groups;
- Comparators: Placebo, no treatment, pharmacotherapies or rehabilitation therapies that are recommended in international clinical practice guidelines;[2–5]
- Outcome measures: Studies reported at least one of the pre-specified outcome measures (Table 4.2).

Exclusion Criteria

- Any case of shoulder complications caused by another clinical condition, such as multiple sclerosis, traumatic brain and spinal cord injuries, etc. were excluded;
- Studies using CM therapies as a comparator;
- In duplicate studies reporting the same results, those published later were excluded.

Outcomes

Included outcomes were determined after consultation with the content expert advisory panel (CEAP) which was convened for this book.

Table 4.2   Pre-specified Outcomes

Outcome Categories	Outcome Measures	Scoring
Motor function	1. FMA motor function	1. Up to 100 points, higher is better
	2. FMA upper limb motor function	2. Up to 66 points, higher is better
	3. FMA lower limb motor function	3. Up to 34 points, higher is better
Activities of daily living	Barthel Index or Modified Barthel Index	Up to 100 points, higher is better
Pain	Pain score visual analogue scale (10 cm)	Up to 100 points, lower is better
Acromiohumeral interval	Acromiohumeral interval	>12 mm
Effective rate	Effective rate	Number of effective cases, from 0% to 100%, higher is better
Adverse events	Number and type of adverse events	

Abbreviations: cm, centimetres; FMA, Fugl-Meyer Assessment; mm, millimetres.

Outcomes of effect included known measures in post-stroke motor function research with a focus on shoulder complications.

Fugl-Meyer Assessment of Motor Recovery after Stroke

The Fugl-Meyer Assessment (FMA) is a disease-specific impairment index designed to assess motor function, balance, sensation qualities and joint function in hemiplegic post-stroke patients.[6,7] The scale comprises five domains: motor function (in the upper and lower extremities), sensory function, balance (both standing and sitting), joint range of motion and joint pain.[8]

Scale items are scored on the basis of ability to complete the item using a 3-point ordinal scale where 0 = cannot perform, 1 = performs partially and 2 = performs fully. The total possible scale score is 226. Points are divided among the domains as follows: 100 points for motor function (66 for upper extremity and 34 for lower extremity), 24 points for sensation (light touch and position sense), 14 points for balance (6 for sitting and 8 for standing), 44 points for joint range of motion (ROM) and 44 points for joint pain. The motor assessment is grounded in well-defined, observable stages of motor recovery.[7]

The FMA is widely used and internationally accepted; it has been used as the gold standard against which the validity of other scales is assessed. Classifications for impairment severity have been proposed based on FMA scores.[9,10]

Placing a specific focus on post-stroke shoulder complications, the FMA upper limb motor function scale (66 points) is reliable in assessing upper extremity function, specifically wrist stability and mobility.

Barthel Index or Modified Barthel Index

The Barthel Index (BI) of activities of daily living (ADL) has been in use since 1955.[11] It was originally intended as a simple index of independence by which to quantify the ability of a patient with a neuromuscular or musculoskeletal disorder to care for him/herself (regardless of particular diagnostic designations). The BI is a simple-to-administer tool for assessing self-care and mobility activities of daily living, consisting of ten common ADL tasks, administered through direct observation. Eight of the ten items represent activities related to personal care; the remaining two are related to mobility. The index yields a total score out of 100 — the higher the score, the greater the degree of functional independence.[12]

Based on the original version of BI, a modified version (Modified Barthel Index, MBI) was introduced by Shah and Vanchay to increase the sensitivity of measurement.[13] This version assessed dependency using scores ranging from 0 (unable to perform task) to a maximum of 5, 10 or 15 (fully independent) for ten domains of functioning (activities): bowel control, bladder control, as well as help with grooming, toilet use, feeding, transfers, walking, dressing, climbing stairs and bathing.[13] The MBI achieved greater sensitivity and improved reliability than the original version, without causing additional difficulty or affecting the implementation time.[13] In addition, another MBI version was also adapted from the original BI scale, which covers the same ten domains but gives a maximum score of 20 (scores ranging from 0 to 2 or 3 for each activity).[14] However, there is a lack of agreement regarding the threshold for in-dependence/dependence, and several different scoring systems are used, making comparisons across groups/studies more difficult.[15]

Visual Analogue Scale

Pain is the primary symptom of post-stroke shoulder complications. The visual analogue scale (VAS) is a commonly used unidimensional measurement instrument to quantify pain intensity.[16] In general, the VAS is used to measure a characteristic or attitude that is believed to range across a continuum of values and cannot easily be directly measured, for example, the amount of pain that a patient feels ranges across a continuum from none to an extreme amount of pain.[17] From the patient's perspective, this spectrum appears continuous and their pain does not take discrete jumps, as a categorisation of none, mild, moderate and severe would suggest. Therefore, the VAS was designed to capture the idea of an underlying continuum.[17]

The pain VAS is a continuous scale comprised of a horizontal (HVAS) or vertical (VVAS) line, usually 10 centimetres (cm, 100 millimetres, mm) in length, anchored by two verbal descriptors, one for each symptom extreme.[18,19]

The pain VAS is self-completed by the respondent. The respondent is asked to place a line perpendicular to the VAS line at the point that represents their pain intensity.[18,20,21] Once the VAS is completed, the assessor can determine the score by measuring the distance on the 10 cm line between the "no pain" anchor and the respondent's mark, providing a range of scores from 0 to 100.

Acromiohumeral Interval

Acromiohumeral interval (AHI) is a useful and reliable measurement on shoulder radiographs. Measurements of the AHI greater than 12 mm suggest a shoulder dislocation or inferior subluxation (e.g. from joint effusion).[22,23]

Shoulder Range of Motion (Range of Shoulder External Rotation)

The normal ROM of a shoulder is defined below for different directions[24]:

- Abduction: 180 degrees;
- Forward flexion: 180 degrees;
- Extension: 60 degrees;
- Rotation:
  - Lateral Rotation: 90 degrees;
  - Medial rotation: 90 degrees.

Among post-stroke patients, the shoulder movement could be impaired, in particular for the shoulder lateral rotation, because it may be the most limited motion in painful stiff shoulders.[25]

Effective Rate

Effective rate was defined as the improvement in clinical symptoms and signs, such as joint swelling, pain and range of shoulder external rotation. The most frequent assessment references were 'Rehabilitation assessment and treatment of stroke 脑卒中的康复评定和治疗',[26] and 'Evaluation and treatment of hemiplegia 偏瘫的现代评价与治疗'.[27] Effectiveness was reported in four levels (clinically cured, remarkably effective, effective and ineffective) or three levels (remarkably effective, effective and ineffective). Effective rate is calculated as the percentage of effective cases of a group. However, there is no standardised definition of 'clinically cured,' 'remarkably effective,' 'effective' and 'ineffective' recommended by clinical guidelines. Considering the non-standardised calculation methods of this outcome, it is only described in the monograph without being used for further synthesis analysis.

Risk of Bias Assessment

Risk of bias was assessed for RCTs using the Cochrane Collaboration's tool.[1] In clinical trials, bias can be categorised as selection bias, performance bias, detection bias, attrition bias and reporting bias. Each domain is assessed to determine whether the bias is at 'low,' 'high' or 'unclear' risk. 'Low' risk of bias indicates that bias is unlikely, 'high' risk indicates plausible bias that seriously weakens confidence in the results and 'unclear' risk of bias indicates lack of information, or uncertainty, over potential bias and raises some doubt about the results. Risk of bias assessment was verified by two people and disagreement was resolved by discussion or consultation with a third person.

Risk of bias is categorised using the following six domains:

- Sequence generation: The method used to generate the allocation sequence is given in sufficient detail to allow an assessment of whether it should produce comparable groups. 'Low' risk of bias refers to a random number table or computer random generator. 'High' risk of bias includes studies that describe a non-random sequence generation such as odd or even date of birth or date of admission;
- Allocation concealment: The method used to conceal the allocation sequence is given in enough detail to determine whether intervention allocations could have been foreseen before, or during, enrolment. 'Low' risk of bias includes central randomisation or sealed envelopes and 'high' risk of bias includes open random sequence or date of birth, etc.;
- Blinding of participants and personnel: These are measures used to describe if the study participants and personnel are blind to the intervention received. In addition, information relating to whether the blinding was effective is also assessed. Studies that ensure blinding of participants and personnel are at 'low' risk of bias. If the study is not blind or is incompletely blind, it is at 'high' risk of bias;
- Blinding of outcome assessors: These are measures used to describe if the outcome assessors are blind to knowledge of which intervention a participant received. In addition, information relating to whether the blinding was effective is also assessed. Studies that ensure blinding of assessors to the outcome are at 'low' risk of

bias. If the study is not blind or is incompletely blind, it is at 'high' risk of bias;

- Incomplete outcome data: This refers to completeness of outcome data for each main outcome, including drop outs, exclusions from the analysis with numbers missing in each group and reasons for drop out or exclusions. Studies with 'low' risk of bias would include all outcome data, or if there is missing data, it is unlikely to relate to the true outcome or is balanced between groups. Studies at 'high' risk of bias would have unexplained missing data;

- Selective reporting: The study protocol is available and the pre-specified outcomes are included in the report. Studies with a published protocol and which include all pre-specified outcomes in their report would be at 'low' risk of bias. Studies at 'high' risk of bias would not include all pre-specified outcomes or the outcome data may be reported incompletely.

Statistical Analyses

Frequency of CM syndromes, CHM formulas, herbs and acupuncture points reported in the included studies are presented using descriptive statistics. CM syndromes reported in two or more studies are presented. The ten most frequently reported CHM formulas and 20 most frequently reported herbs are presented and where used in at least two studies, although for CHM formulas this was not always possible. The top ten acupuncture points used in two or more studies are presented, or as available. Where data was limited, reports of single CM syndromes or acupuncture points are provided as a guide for the reader.

Definitions of statistical tests and results are described in the glossary. Dichotomous data are reported as a risk ratio (RR) with 95% confidence intervals (CI), and continuous data are reported as mean difference (MD) or standard mean difference (SMD) with 95% CI. For all analyses, RR, MD or SMD together with 95% CI were reported, as well as a formal test for heterogeneity using the I^2 statistic. An I^2 score greater than 50% was considered to indicate substantial heterogeneity.[1] Sensitivity analyses were undertaken to explore potential sources of heterogeneity, based on low risk of bias for one of the risk of bias domains, sequence generation. Where possible and appropriate, planned subgroup analyses included duration of disease or treatment, CM syndromes, CHM formulas and comparator type. Available case analysis with a random effects model was used in all analyses. The random effects model was used to take into account the clinical heterogeneity likely to be encountered within, and between, included studies, and the variation in treatment effects between included studies.

Assessment Using GRADE

The Grading of Recommendations Assessment, Development and Evaluation (GRADE) approach was used.[28] The GRADE approach summarises and rates the strength and quality (certainty) of evidence in systematic reviews using a structured process for presenting evidence summaries. The results are presented in 'summary of findings' tables. The results provide an important overview for post-stroke spasticity outcomes.

A panel of experts was established to evaluate the quality of evidence. The panel included the systematic review team, CM practitioners, integrative medicine experts, research methodologists and conventional medicine physicians. The experts were asked to rate the clinical importance of key interventions from CHM, acupuncture therapies and other CM therapies as well as comparators and outcomes. Results were collated, and based on the rating scores and subsequent discussion, a consensus on the contents for the 'summary of findings' tables was achieved.

The certainty of evidence for each outcome was rated according to five factors outlined in the GRADE approach. The certainty of evidence may be rated based on:

- Limitations in study design (risk of bias);
- Inconsistency of results (unexplained heterogeneity);
- Indirectness of evidence (interventions, populations and outcomes important to the patients with the condition);
- Imprecision (uncertainty about the results);
- Publication bias (selective publication of studies).

These five factors are additive and a reduction in more than one factor will reduce the certainty of the evidence for that outcome. The GRADE approach also includes three domains that can be rated up, including large magnitude of an effect, dose-response gradient and effect of plausible residual confounding. However, these three domains relate to observational studies including cohort, case-control, before-after, time-series studies, etc. GRADE summaries in this book only include RCTs, therefore these three domains for rating up were not assessed.

Treatment recommendations can also be assessed using the GRADE approach but due to the diverse nature of CM practice, treatment recommendations were not included with the summary of findings. Therefore, the reader is able to interpret the evidence with reference to the local practice environment. It should also be noted that the GRADE approach requires judgments about the quality of evidence and some subjective assessment. However, the experience of the panel members suggests the judgments are reliable and transparent representations of the certainty of evidence.

The GRADE levels of evidence are grouped into four categories:

1. 'High' certainty: Further research is very unlikely to change our confidence in the estimate of effect;
2. 'Moderate' certainty: Further research is likely to have an important impact on our confidence in the estimate of effect and may change the estimate;
3. 'Low' certainty: Further research is very likely to have an important impact on our confidence in the estimate of effect and is likely to change the estimate;
4. 'Very low' certainty: Any estimate of effect is very uncertain.

References

1. Higgins J, Green S, eds. (2011) *Cochrane Handbook for Systematic Reviews of Interventions Version 5.1.0.* The Cochrane Collaboration. Available from: http://www.cochrane-handbook.org.

2. Duncan PW, Zorowitz R, Bates B, *et al.* (2005) Management of adult stroke rehabilitation care: A clinical practice guideline. *Stroke* **36**(9): e100–e143.

3. Mehta S, Teasull R, Foley N. (last updated 2018) Evidence-based review of stroke rehabilitation: Painful hemiplegic shoulder. Available from: http://www.ebrsr.com/evidence-review/11-hemiplegic-shoulder-pain-complex-regional-pain-syndrome.

4. Paci M, Nannetti L, Rinaldi LA. (2005) Glenohumeral subluxation in hemiplegia: An overview. *J Rehabil Res Dev* **42**(4): 557–568.

5. Winstein CJ, Stein J, Arena R, *et al.* (2016) Guidelines for adult stroke rehabilitation and recovery: A guideline for healthcare professionals from the American Heart Association/American Stroke Association. American Heart Association Stroke Council, Council on Cardiovascular and Stroke Nursing, Council on Clinical Cardiology, and Council on Quality of Care and Outcomes Research. *Stroke* **47**(6): e98–e169.

6. Fugl-Meyer AR, Jaasko L, Leyman I, *et al.* (1975) The post-stroke hemiplegic patient. 1. A method for evaluation of physical performance. *Scand J Rehabil Med* **7**(1): 13–31.

7. Gladstone DJ, Danells CJ, Black SE. (2002) The Fugl-Meyer assessment of motor recovery after stroke: A critical review of its measurement properties. *Neurorehabil Neural Repair* **16**(3): 232–240.

8. Chae, J, Labatia I, Yang G. (2003) Upper limb motor function in hemiparesis: Concurrent validity of the Arm Motor Ability test. *Am J Phys Med Rehabil* **82**(1): 1–8.

9. Duncan PW, Goldstein LB, Horner RD, *et al.* (1994) Similar motor recovery of upper and lower extremities after stroke. *Stroke* **25**(6): 1181–1188.

10. Fugl-Meyer AR. (1980) Post-stroke hemiplegia assessment of physical properties. *Scand J Rehabil Med Suppl* (7): 85–93.

11. Mahoney FI. (1965) Functional evaluation: The Barthel Index. *MD State Med J* **14**: 61–65.

12. McDowell I. (2006) *Measuring Health: A Guide to Rating Scales and Questionnaires*, 3rd ed. Oxford University Press. Available from: https://www.fundacion-salto.org/documentos/Measuring%20Health.pdf.

13. Shah S, Vanclay F, Cooper B. (1989) Improving the sensitivity of the Barthel Index for stroke rehabilitation. *J Clin Epidemiol* **42**: 703–709.

14. Collin C, Wade DT, Davies S, Horne V. (1988) The Barthel ADL Index: A reliability study. *Int Disabil Stud* **10**(2): 61–63.

15. Quinn TJ, Langhorne P, Stott DJ. (2011) Barthel Index for stroke trials: Development, properties, and application. *Stroke* **42**(4): 1146–1151.
16. McCormack HM, Horne DJ, Sheather S. (1988) Clinical applications of visual analogue scales: A critical review. *Psychol Med* **18**: 1007–1019.
17. Gould D. Visual Analogue Scale (VAS). (2001) *J Clin Nurs* **10**: 697–706.
18. Huskisson EC. (1974) Measurement of pain. *Lancet* **2**: 1127–1131.
19. Jensen MP, Karoly P, Braver S. (1986) The measurement of clinical pain intensity: A comparison of six methods. *Pain* **27**: 117–126.
20. Scott J, Huskisson EC. (1976) Graphic representation of pain. *Pain* **2**: 175–184.
21. Joyce CR, Zutshi DW, Hrubes VF, Mason RM. (1975) Comparison of fixed interval and visual analogue scales for rating chronic pain. *Eur J Clin Pharmacol* **8**: 415–420.
22. Gruber G, Bernhardt GA, Clar H, *et al.* (2010) Measurement of the acromiohumeral interval on standardized anteroposterior radiographs: A prospective study of observer variability. *J Shoulder Elbow Surg* **19**(1): 10–13.
23. Davies AM, ed. (2004) *Imaging of the Shoulder: Techniques and Applications (Medical Radiology/Diagnostic Imaging)*. Springer, New York.
24. 卓大宏. (2003) 中国康复医学, 2nd ed. Hua Xia Publishing House, Beijing.
25. Andrews AW, Bohannon RW. (1989) Decreased shoulder range of motion on paretic side after stroke. *Phys Ther* **69**(9): 768–772.
26. 缪鸿石, 朱镛连. (1996) Rehabilitation assessment and treatment of stroke 脑卒中的康复评定和治疗. Hua Xia Publishing House, Beijing.
27. 王茂斌. (1990) Evaluation and treatment of hemiplegia 偏瘫的现代评价与治疗. Hua Xia Publishing House, Beijing.
28. Schunemann H, Brozek J, Guyatt G, Oxman A, eds. (2013) *GRADE Handbook for Grading Quality of Evidence and Strength of Recommendations*. The GRADE Working Group. Available from: http://www.guidelinedevelopment.org/handbook/.

5

Clinical Evidence for Chinese Herbal Medicine

OVERVIEW

This chapter evaluates the available clinical evidence for Chinese herbal medicine for its effects on post-stroke shoulder disorders. Where appropriate, Chinese herbal medicine treatments are pooled together in a meta-analysis to assess their overall effect for shoulder sublaxation, shoulder pain and shoulder-hand syndrome. The quality of evidence is also evaluated to assess the strength of available data.

Introduction

Chinese herbal medicine (CHM) has been examined by many studies which have been published in scientific journals, both in China and internationally. A rigorous screening process was undertaken to identify clinical studies of CHM for the treatment of three common post-stroke shoulder conditions: (1) shoulder subluxation; (2) shoulder pain and (3) shoulder-hand syndrome (SHS). These studies included randomised controlled trials (RCTs), non-randomised controlled clinical trials (CCTs) and non-controlled studies. Evidence from RCTs has been pooled to evaluate the efficacy and safety of CHM alone, or in combination with conventional therapy for post-stroke shoulder disorders. CCTs were evaluated using the same approach as for RCTs, and are described separately. Evidence from non-controlled studies is more difficult to evaluate, therefore the approach was taken to describe the characteristics of the study, details of the intervention and any adverse events. The findings of the literature search are presented in this chapter.

Identification of Clinical Studies

Search of nine English and Chinese language databases identified 37,141 citations, of which, 1,096 required full text retrieval to determine their eligibility for inclusion (Fig. 5.1). After assessment against rigorous inclusion criteria, 83 clinical studies which evaluated CHM for post-stroke shoulder complications were included. Seventy studies were RCTs, two were non-randomised CCTs, and 11 were non-controlled studies. Of these, 20 studies evaluated oral CHM, 59 studies assessed topical CHM and four studies were of the combination of oral CHM and topical CHM. More details and treatment results of CHM for three post-stroke shoulder complications are presented below separately. Controlled studies (RCTs and CCTs) were evaluated to assess the efficacy and safety of CHM for post-stroke shoulder complications, and details from non-controlled studies are described.

In addition, one study was identified utilising interventions not commonly practised outside of China; this study was not presented here.

Shoulder Subluxation

For stroke patients, if insufficient support and therapy are provided to the shoulder, subluxation of shoulder joint may result. The clinical intention of post-stroke care is typically to prevent shoulder subluxation; however, if it develops the disorder can lead to shoulder pain and for severe cases it can lead to SHS. No studies were found that utilised oral CHM for subluxation, while topical CHM therapies seem the preferred intervention.

Topical Chinese Herbal Medicine

Two RCTs (H1, H2) and one non-controlled study (H4) were found using topical CHM for subluxation.

Records identified through Chinese language database searching
($n = 28,818$)

Records identified through English language database searching
($n = 8,316$)

Records identified through other sources
($n = 7$)

Records after duplicates removed English database ($n = 22,597$)

Records screened ($n = 22,597$)

Records excluded ($n = 21,501$)

Full-text articles assessed for eligibility ($n = 1,096$)

Full-text articles excluded, with reasons ($n = 1,013$):
• Duplicates in Chinese databases ($n = 85$);
• Not clinical studies ($n = 115$);
• Not Chinese medicine ($n = 40$);
• Not treating post-stroke shoulder complications ($n = 205$);
• Not meeting the inclusion criteria ($n = 254$);
• Did not provide data ($n = 51$);
• Not CHM as intervention ($n = 262$);
• CHM therapy not included in this book ($n = 1$).

Non-controlled studies
($n = 11$)

Non-randomised controlled trials
($n = 2$)

Randomised controlled trials
($n = 70$)

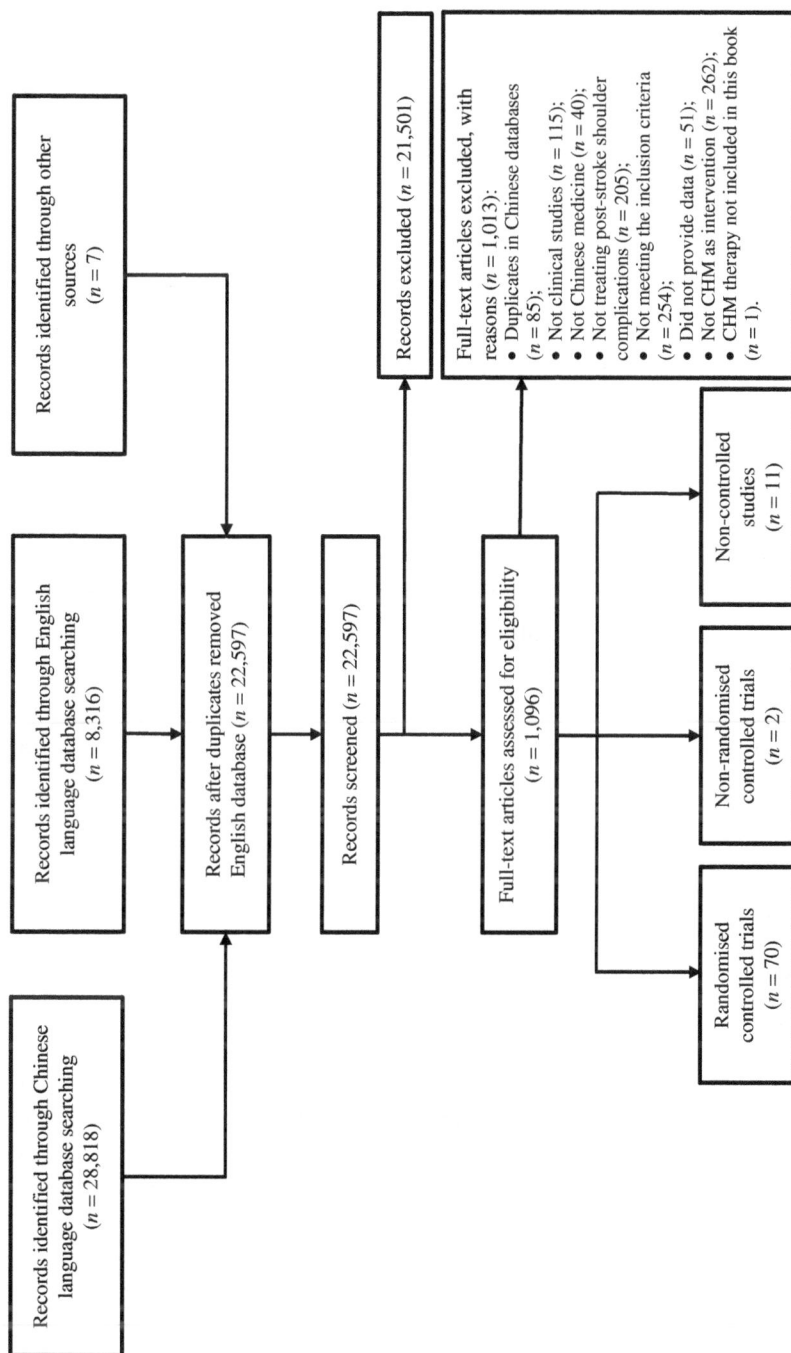

Fig. 5.1 Flowchart of study selection process: Chinese herbal medicine.

Randomised Controlled Trials of Topical Chinese Herbal Medicine

Two RCTs evaluated topical CHM for post-stroke shoulder sublaxation; neither of the studies named their formulas. One study (H1) used CHM steam therapy (ingredients: *wei ling xian* 威灵仙, *chuan xiong* 川芎, *niu xi* 牛膝, *tou gu cao* 透骨草, *fang feng* 防风, *gui zhi* 桂枝, *ai ye* 艾叶, *shen jin cao* 伸筋草, *hai zao* 海藻, *kun bu* 昆布, *hong hua* 红花, *dang gui* 当归, *zhi cao wu* 制草乌 and *zhi chuan wu* 制川乌). The other study (H2) used CHM fomentation (ingredients: *xu duan* 续断, *du zhong* 杜仲, *niu xi* 牛膝, *tian qi* 田七, *qiang huo* 羌活, *du huo* 独活, *tao ren* 桃仁, *hong hua* 红花, *gu sui bu* 骨碎补, *shen jin cao* 伸筋草, *bai shao* 白芍 and *qi ye yi zhi hua* 七叶一枝花). Neither study reported the same outcome, with activities of daily living (ADL) assessed by Modified Barthel Index (MBI) and pain visual analogue scale (VAS) reported by one study (H1), and Fugl-Meyer Assessment (FMA) reported by the other study (H2). One study (H1) included 62 subjects with a greater effect in the CHM group compared to the control group for both MBI: mean difference (MD: 10.20 [7.97, 12.43]) and pain VAS (MD: –1.20 [–1.81, –0.59]) at the end of treatment. For the other study (H2), of the 71 participants, it also favoured the integration of CHM and rehabilitation compared to rehabilitation alone for FMA (MD: 14.85 [12.66, 17.04]).

Risk of Bias

One study (H1) was rated 'low' risk for sequence generation as it used a random number table, whilst the other RCT (H2) was rated as 'unclear' because insufficient details were reported. For remaining items, both studies were rated the same; 'high' risk of bias for participant and personnel blinding as blinding methods were not utilised; 'unclear' risk for blinding of assessors as there was insufficient information to provide a rating. For incomplete outcome reporting both studies were assessed as 'low' risk, and for selective reporting both were rated 'unclear' as neither study was registered or reported a published protocol to evaluate their outcome reporting.

Assessment Using GRADE

At the conclusion of a consensus process as described in Chapter 4, it was determined that summary of findings tables should be prepared for the comparison of topical CHM combined with routine rehabilitation vs. rehabilitation alone. Two studies compared topical CHM as integrative medicine with routine rehabilitation (H1, H2), with one study (H2) reporting data on FMA and another study reporting data on ADL and pain VAS (H1). Shoulder range of motion (ROM) and adverse events were not reported by these studies. Evidence for topical CHM as integrative medicine with routine rehabilitation for three outcomes is 'low' certainty, although significant benefit of adding topical CHM was found (Table 5.1).

Non-controlled Clinical Studies of Topical Chinese Herbal Medicine

Only one non-controlled clinical study (H4) evaluated topical CHM for shoulder subluxation. It utilised CHM steam therapy in 96 people and combined CHM with usual care rehabilitative therapies. The study also allowed for acupuncture and pharmacotherapy use. The name of the study's CHM formulas or the ingredients was not reported. Outcome measures reported included FMA, pain VAS and effective rate. No adverse events were reported.

Shoulder Pain

Following subluxation, sufferers can experience pain requiring clinical intervention to reduce the pain and improve the ROM to the shoulder. Therapy is aimed at reducing local pain and inflammation, encouraging blood flow to the area and freeing up movement.

Oral Chinese Herbal Medicine for Shoulder Pain

Likely due to the local nature of shoulder pain, only one study (H5) utilised oral CHM for shoulder pain. The study was an RCT which inves-

Table 5.1   GRADE: Topical Chinese Herbal Medicine Plus Routine Rehabilitation vs. Routine Rehabilitation for Post-stroke Shoulder Subluxation

Outcomes	No of Participants (Studies) Follow-up	Certainty of the Evidence (GRADE)	Anticipated Absolute Effects	
			Risk with Rehabilitation	Risk Difference with Topical CHM + Rehabilitation
FMA	71 (1 RCT)	⊕⊕⊖⊖ LOW[a,b]	The mean FMA was **22.41**	MD **14.85 higher** (12.66 higher to 17.04 higher)
ADL	62 (1 RCT)	⊕⊕⊖⊖ LOW[a,b]	The mean ADL was **75.6**	MD **10.2 higher** (7.97 higher to 12.43 higher)
Pain VAS	62 (1 RCT)	⊕⊕⊖⊖ LOW[a,b]	The mean VAS was **3.1**	MD **1.2 lower** (1.81 lower to 0.59 lower)

The risk in the intervention group (and its 95% confidence interval) is based on the assumed risk in the comparison group and the relative effect of the intervention (and its 95% CI).

Abbreviations: ADL, activities of daily living; CHM, Chinese herbal medicine; CI, confidence interval; FMA, Fugl-Meyer Assessment; GRADE, Grading of Recommendations Assessment, Development and Evaluation; MD, mean difference; RCT, randomised control trial; VAS, visual analogue scale.

Notes:

a. Lack of blinding of participants, personnel and assessors.
b. Small sample size limits certainty of results.

Study References:

FMA: H2
ADL: H1
Pain VAS: H1

tigated modified *Shen tong zhu yu tang* 身痛逐瘀汤 combined with rehabilitation (n = 35) compared to pharmacotherapy (IV oxerutins 800 mg once a day and ibuprofen 300 mg twice a day) plus rehabilitation therapy (n = 33). The study reported greater effects for ADL assessed by Bathel Index (BI) (MD: 15.76 [14.20, 17.32]) and pain score (MD: −2.07 [−2.48, −1.66]) in the CHM group, with no adverse events reported. Oxerutins is a venoactive drug indicated for venous insufficiency[1] whilst ibuprofen is commonly used for inflammation and pain.

Topical Chinese Herbal Medicine for Shoulder Pain

Fifteen studies investigated topical forms of CHM for shoulder pain; 12 (H6–H17) were RCTs, one (H3) was a non-randomised CCT and two (H18, H19) were non-controlled studies.

Randomised Controlled Trials of Topical Chinese Herbal Medicine

A total of 12 RCTs evaluated topical CHM in 937 people. Duration of the intervention for the studies ranged between 10 days (H6, H7) and two months (H8). Of those studies reporting participant gender, more males (n = 291) over females (n = 256) were included. Six studies (H6, H9–H13) evaluated CHM fomentation and the other six (H7, H8, H14–H17) used CHM steam therapy.

Of the CHM fomentation studies (H6, H9–H13), all were integrated and compared with rehabilitation. One study (H9) also utilised computerised intermediate frequency therapy in both the intervention and control arms. All the CHM steam therapy studies (H7, H8, H14–H17) also integrated CHM with rehabilitation, except for one study of 49 people which utilised a neurodevelopment therapy known as Bobath movement therapy (H14). One study of 80 people (H7), in addition to CHM and rehabilitation therapy, also added thermal magnetic therapy and ultrashort wave electrotherapy. It was noted that two CHM fomentation publications likely reported the same study results so their data were merged together (H12, H13).

Table 5.2   Frequently Reported Topically Used Herbs in Randomised Controlled Trials for Shoulder Pain

Most Common Herbs	Scientific Name	No. of Studies
Chuan xiong 川芎	*Ligusticum chuangxiong* Hort.	8
Hong hua 红花	*Carthamus tinctorius* L.	8
Tou gu cao 透骨草	Herba Clematidis Intricatae	8
Wei ling xian 威灵仙	*Clematis chinensis* Osbeck/*Clematis hexapetala* Pall./ *Clematis manshurica* Rupr.	7
Dang gui 当归	*Angelica sinensis* Oliv. Diels	5
Gui zhi 桂枝	*Cinnamomum cassia* Presl	5
Shen jin cao 伸筋草	*Lycopodium japonicum* Thunb.	4
Wu tou 乌头	*Aconitum carmichaelii* Debx.	4
Chi shao 赤芍	*Paeonia lactiflora* Pall./*Paeonia veitchii* Lynch	3
Mo yao 没药	*Commiphora myrrha* Engl./*Commiphora molmol* Engl.	3
Mu gua 木瓜	*Chaenomeles speciosa* Sweet Nakai	3
Ru xiang 乳香	*Boswellia carterii* Birdw./*Boswellia bhaw-dajiana* Birdw.	3

Note: The use of some herbs such as *wu tou* 乌头 may be restricted in some countries. Readers are advised to comply with relevant regulations.

Only one study (H9) reported the formula name used, *Gu ci xiao tong ye* 骨刺消痛液. None of the 12 studies reported Chinese medicine syndrome type. See Table 5.2 for the most common herbs.

Risk of Bias

Four of the included RCTs (H6, H8, H12, H13) were rated as 'low' risk of bias for sequence generation, with the remaining eight evaluated as 'unclear' risk due to insufficient reporting. All 12 RCTs were assessed 'unclear' risk for allocation concealment again due to insufficient reporting, whilst for blinding of participants and personnel they were rated 'high' risk as blinding methods were not employed. The blinding of outcome assessors for all RCTs was of 'unclear' risk as reported information was insufficient to make a clear judgment.

Table 5.3   Risk of Bias of Randomised Controlled Trials: Topical Chinese Herbal Medicine for Shoulder Pain

Risk of Bias Domain	Low Risk n (%)	Unclear Risk n (%)	High Risk n (%)
Sequence generation	4 (33.3)	9 (67)	0
Allocation concealment	0	12 (100)	0
Blinding of participants	0	0	12 (100)
Blinding of personnel	0	0	12 (100)
Blinding of outcome assessors	0	12 (100)	0
Incomplete outcome data	12 (100)	0	0
Selective outcome reporting	0	11 (91.6)	1 (8.3)

None of the studies had incomplete data so were all rated as 'low' risk for this. Only one of the studies (H12) was evaluated to be 'high' risk for selective outcome reporting. In the methods section of the publication it stated it would report safety data, yet the results section did not report it. The other 11 studies were rated 'unclear' risk as they did not report publication or registration of their protocol. See Table 5.3 for details.

Outcomes for Shoulder Pain

Main outcomes reported by the included studies consisted of FMA, ADL, pain VAS and effective rate. The pain VAS (H6–H8, H10, H12, H14, H15) and effective rate (H7, H9–H12, H16, H17) were most commonly reported, each by seven studies, whilst the FMA was reported by six (H7–H10, H12, H15) and the ADL assessed by BI was reported by two studies (H6, H10). Only one study (H10) reported all these outcome measures. For each of the outcome measures a subgroup analysis of studies was conducted based on their topical form of CHM, either fomentation or CHM steam therapy.

Effects of topical Chinese herbal medicine for shoulder pain

The effects of topical CHM for treating shoulder pain are presented below under each outcome measures. Table 5.4 summarises the

Table 5.4 Topical Chinese Herbal Medicine as Integrative Medicine vs. Rehabilitation Therapy: Shoulder Pain

Outcome	No. of Studies	No. of Participants	Effect Size (MD [95% CI])	I² %	Included Studies
FMA	6	564	7.59 [3.53, 11.65]*	95	H7–H10, H12, H15
ADL (BI)	2	204	8.89 [4.15, 13.62]*	0	H6, H10
Pain score or VAS	7	472	−1.54 [−2.07, −1.01]*	83	H6–H8, H10, H12, H14, H15

*Statistically significant. Abbreviations: ADL, activities of daily living; BI, Bathel Index; CI, confidence interval; FMA, Fugl-Meyer Assessment; MD, mean difference; VAS, visual analogue scale.

Table 5.5 Topical Chinese Herbal Medicine as Integrative Medicine for Shoulder Pain Subgroup Analyses

Intervention	Outcome	No. of Studies	No. of Participants	Effect Size (MD [95% CI])	I² %	Included Studies
Fomentation	FMA	3	304	5.45 [1.36, 9.55]*	83	H9, H10, H12
	Pain score or VAS	3	264	−1.05 [−1.54, −0.56]*	52	H6, H10, H12
Steam therapy	FMA	3	260	9.43 [5.07, 13.78]*	91	H7, H8, H15
	Pain score or VAS	4	308	−1.87 [−2.70, −1.04]*	87	H7, H8, H14, H15

*Statistically significant. Abbreviations: CI, confidence interval; FMA, Fugl-Meyer Assessment; MD, mean difference; VAS, visual analogue scale.

overall meta-analyses results and Table 5.5 lists the subgroups meta-analyses results.

Fugl-Meyer Assessment

There were no topical CHM-alone RCTs which used FMA as an outcome. For RCTs integrating CHM with conventional therapy, seven publications for six studies reported FMA in a total of 564 people (H7–H10, H12, H15; Note: H12 and H13 referred to the same study).

These RCTs were combined in a meta-analysis, the results indicating the combination of topical CHM and rehabilitation therapy was more effective than rehabilitation alone for shoulder pain (MD: 7.59 [3.53, 11.65], $I^2 = 95\%$).

Studies were subgrouped according to their topical application form. Three studies (H9, H10, H12) utilised CHM as fomentation integrated with rehabilitation therapies and showed an improved effect compared to rehabilitation therapy alone (MD: 5.45 [1.36, 9.55], $I^2 = 83\%$). For the three studies (H7, H8, H15) utilising steam therapy, again CHM integrated with rehabilitation had a greater effect (MD: 9.43 [5.07, 13.78], $I^2 = 91\%$).

Pain Score or Visual Analogue Scale

Seven RCTs involving 472 people (H6–H8, H10, H12, H14, H15) integrated topical CHM and some form of rehabilitation therapy and reported pain score or pain VAS as an outcome measure for shoulder pain. Meta-analysis of these studies favoured the combination of topical CHM and rehabilitation therapy (MD: –1.54 [–2.07, –1.01], $I^2 = 83\%$).

Activities of Daily Living (Bathel Index)

There were no RCTs of topical CHM alone for shoulder pain. Two studies (H6, H10) assessed BI as an outcome measure in 204 people with both studies utilising fomentation form of CHM. Meta-analysis favoured integrating CHM fomentation with rehabilitative therapy (MD: 8.89 [4.15, 13.62], $I^2 = 0\%$).

Effective Rate

Seven studies integrating topical CHM with rehabilitation therapy utilised some form of effective rate as an outcome in 569 people (H7, H9–H12, H16, H17). As their measure of effective rate varied between these studies they were not pooled in a meta-analysis.

Assessment Using GRADE

As the result of our consensus process, a summary of findings table was prepared for the comparison of topical CHM combined with routine rehabilitation vs. rehabilitation alone. Six studies (H7–H10, H12, H15) reported data on FMA, two studies (H6, H10) reported ADL and seven studies (H6–H8, H10, H12, H14, H15) reported pain score or VAS. Evidence for topical CHM as integrative medicine with routine rehabilitation for these three outcomes is 'low' or 'very low' certainty, although significant benefit of adding topical CHM was found in all meta-analyses or subgroup meta-analyses (Table 5.6).

Randomised Controlled Trial Evidence for Individual Topical Formulas

Only one RCT (H9) reported the name of its CHM formula: *Gu ci xiao tong ye* 骨刺消痛液 (containing the herbs *chuan wu* 川乌, *cao wu* 草乌, *ma huang* 麻黄, *gui zhi* 桂枝, *du huo* 独活, *tie si wei ling xian* 铁丝威灵仙, *hong hua* 红花, *dang gui* 当归, *chuan xiong* 川芎, *wu mei* 乌梅, *mu gua* 木瓜 and *niu xi* 牛膝). From Chapter 2, there is little guidance and recommendation for topical therapy for shoulder pain, with the 'CHM Compound to Free Collateral Vessels Decoction 复方通络液' as CHM steam therapy being the only formula with potential indication. This formula has four herbs in common with the previous mentioned formula, *Gu ci xiao tong ye* 骨刺消痛液; they are *chuan wu* 川乌, *hong hua* 红花, *dang gui* 当归 and *chuan xiong* 川芎. Both formulas function to move Blood stasis, free the flow of the collaterals and reduce pain.

Frequently Reported Topically Used Herbs in Meta-analyses Showing Favourable Effect for Shoulder Pain

The most frequently reported herbs from studies favouring integration of topical CHM for shoulder pain were calculated and are presented in Table 5.7. Frequency is grouped according to outcome measures (FMA, ADL, pain score or VAS), regardless of the form of CHM intervention (steam therapy or fomentation).

Table 5.6 GRADE: Topical Chinese Herbal Medicine Plus Routine Rehabilitation vs. Routine Rehabilitation for Post-stroke Shoulder Pain

Outcomes	No. of Participants (Studies) Follow-up	Certainty of the Evidence (GRADE)	Anticipated Absolute Effects	
			Risk with Rehabilitation	Risk Difference with Topical CHM + Rehabilitation
FMA	564 (6 RCTs)	⊕⊕◯◯ LOW[a,b]	The mean FMA was **24.21**	MD **7.59 higher** (3.53 higher to 11.65 higher)
FMA — fomentation	304 (3 RCTs)	⊕◯◯◯ VERY LOW[a,b,c]	The mean FMA — fomentation was **26.63**	MD **5.45 higher** (1.36 higher to 9.55 higher)
FMA — steam	260 (3 RCTs)	⊕◯◯◯ VERY LOW[a,b,c]	The mean FMA — steam was **21.33**	MD **9.43 higher** (5.07 higher to 13.78 higher)
ADL — fomentation	204 (2 RCTs)	⊕⊕◯◯ LOW[a,b]	The mean ADL (fomentation only) was **55.58**	MD **8.89 higher** (4.15 higher to 13.62 higher)
Pain score or VAS	572 (7 RCTs)	⊕⊕◯◯ LOW[a,c]	The mean VAS was **3.82**	MD **1.54 lower** (2.07 lower to 1.01 lower)
Pain score or VAS — steam	264 (3 RCTs)	⊕⊕◯◯ LOW[a,b]	The mean VAS — steam was **3.73**	MD **1.05 lower** (1.54 lower to 0.56 lower)

(Continued)

Table 5.6 *(Continued)*

Outcomes	No. of Participants (Studies) Follow-up	Certainty of the Evidence (GRADE)	Anticipated Absolute Effects	
			Risk with Rehabilitation	Risk Difference with Topical CHM + Rehabilitation
Pain score or VAS — fomentation	308 (4 RCTs)	⊕◯◯◯ VERY LOW[a,b,c]	The mean VAS — Fumigation was **3.89**	MD **1.87 lower** (2.7 lower to 1.04 lower)
Adverse events	80 (1 RCT)	The study reported there was no adverse event observed.		

The risk in the intervention group (and its 95% confidence interval) is based on the assumed risk in the comparison group and the relative effect of the intervention (and its 95% CI).

Abbreviations: ADL, activities of daily living; CHM, Chinese herbal medicine; CI, confidence interval; FMA, Fugl-Meyer Assessment; GRADE, Grading of Recommendations Assessment, Development and Evaluation; MD, mean difference; RCT, randomised control trial; VAS, visual analogue scale.

Note:

a. Lack of blinding of participants and personnel.
b. Considerable statistical heterogeneity.
c. Small sample size limits certainty of results.

Study References

FMA: H7–H10, H12, H15
FMA — fomentation: H9, H10, H12
FMA — steam: H7, H8, H15
ADL (fomentation only): H6, H10
Pain score or VAS: H6–H8, H10, H12, H14, H15
Pain score or VAS — steam: H6, H10, H12
Pain score or VAS — fomentation: H7, H8, H14, H15
Adverse events: H7

Table 5.7 Frequently Reported Topically Used Herbs in Meta-analyses Showing Favourable Effect for Shoulder Pain: Fomentation and Chinese Herbal Medicine Steam Therapy

Outcome Measure	No. of Meta-analyses	No. of Studies	Herbs	Scientific Name	No. of Studies Using Herb
FMA	2	6	Chuan xiong 川芎	*Ligusticum chuangxiong* Hort.	6
			Wei ling xian 威灵仙	*Clematis chinensis* Osbeck/ *Clematis hexapetala* Pall./ *Clematis manshurica* Rupr.	4
			Gui zhi 桂枝	*Cinnamomum cassia* Presl	4
			Hong hua 红花	*Carthamus tinctorius* L.	4
			Tou gu cao 透骨草	Herba Clematidis Intricatae	4
			Dang gui 当归	*Angelica sinensis* (Oliv.) Diels	3
			Chi shao 赤芍	*Paeonia lactiflora* Pall./ *Paeonia veitchii* Lynch	2
			Ru xiang 乳香	*Boswellia carterii* Birdw./ *Boswellia bhaw-dajiana* Birdw.	2
			Mo yao 没药	*Commiphora myrrha* Engl./ *Commiphora molmol* Engl.	2
			Yan hu suo 延胡索	*Corydalis yanhusuo* W. T. Wang	2
ADL	1	2	Chuan xiong 川芎	*Ligusticum chuangxiong* Hort.	2
			Hong hua 红花	*Carthamus tinctorius* L.	2
			Chi shao 赤芍	*Paeonia lactiflora* Pall./ *Paeonia veitchii* Lynch	2
			Ai ye 艾叶	*Artemisia argyi* Lévl. et Vant.	2
Pain VAS	2	7	Chuan xiong 川芎	*Ligusticum chuangxiong* Hort.	6
			Hong hua cao 红花	*Carthamus tinctorius* L.	4
			Wei ling xian 威灵仙	*Clematis chinensis* Osbeck/ *Clematis hexapetala* Pall./ *Clematis manshurica* Rupr.	4
			Tou gu cao 透骨草	Herba Clematidis Intricatae	4
			Dang gui 当归	*Angelica sinensis* (Oliv.) Diels	3

(Continued)

Table 5.7   (Continued)

Outcome Measure	No. of Meta-analyses	No. of Studies	Herbs	Scientific Name	No. of Studies Using Herb
			Chi shao 赤芍	*Paeonia lactiflora* Pall./ *Paeonia veitchii* Lynch	3
			Gui zhi 桂枝	*Cinnamomum cassia* Presl	3
			Shen jin cao 伸筋草	*Lycopodium japonicum* Thunb.	2
			Yan hu suo 延胡索	*Corydalis yanhusuo* W. T. Wang	2
			Ru xiang 乳香	*Boswellia carterii* Birdw./ *Boswellia bhaw-dajiana* Birdw.	2
			Mo yao 没药	*Commiphora myrrha* Engl./ *Commiphora molmol* Engl.	2

Abbreviations: ADL, activities of daily living; FMA, Fugl-Meyer Assessment; VAS, visual analogue scale.

Controlled Clinical Trials (Non-randomised) of Topical Chinese Herbal Medicine

One non-randomised CCT (H3) reported using a topical CHM for shoulder pain. The study used *Si zi san* 四子散 (containing *su zi* 苏子, *lai fu zi* 莱菔子, *bai jie zi* 白芥子and *wu zhu yu* 吴茱萸), administered using fomentation, twice daily for three weeks alongside rehabilitation therapy. It reported FMA (MD: 32.37 [23.71, 41.03]), BI (MD: 23.68 [15.70, 31.66]) and pain VAS (MD: −1.92 [−2.68, −1.16]); all had superior improvement with integration of topical CHM with rehabilitation (*n* = 30) compared to rehabilitation alone (*n* = 30).

Non-controlled Clinical Studies of Topical Chinese Herbal Medicine

Two studies used topical CHM for shoulder pain in 70 people. One study (H18), reporting only effective rate, administered CHM fomentation in 30 people along with rehabilitation using an unnamed formula (contaning *wu zhu yu* 吴茱萸, *tu si zi* 菟丝子, *lai fu zi* 莱菔子, *dong kui zi* 冬葵子 and *bai jie zi* 白芥子). The other study (H19), reporting shoulder ROM and pain scores in 40 people, externally applied CHM along with movement therapy also using an unnamed formula (containing *dan shen* 丹参, *ru xiang* 乳香, *mo yao* 没药, *wu ling zhi* 五灵脂, *pu huang* 蒲黄, *san qi* 三七, *bing pian* 冰片, *tou gu cao* 透骨草 and *shen jin cao* 伸筋草).

Controlled and Non-controlled Clinical Trial Evidence for Individual Topical Formula

The formula *Si zi san* 四子散 (H3) does not correspond to Chapter 2 review of literature and its contained herbal ingredients are also not in the list of most frequently used topical herbs for fomentation or CHM steam therapy. More research into this formula is needed to evaluate its effectiveness, compared to other recommended CHM formulas for shoulder pain. More published reporting of formula name by studies is needed to evaluate any superiority of a particular CHM formulation, and formula section should consider recommended guidelines and textbooks.

Shoulder-hand Syndrome

Oral Chinese Herbal Medicine for Shoulder-hand Syndrome

As SHS is a more chronic shoulder disorder, clinically it may require both local and internal treatment. Oral CHM studies were most frequent for this shoulder disorder than for the others. A total of 17 RCTs and two non-controlled studies was found which evaluated oral CHM.

Randomised Controlled Trials of Oral Chinese Herbal Medicine

In total 17 RCTs (H20–H36) investigated oral CHM for SHS in 1,441 people, although two studies (H29, H35) contained additional control arm data which were excluded from analysis. Of the studies reporting

Table 5.8   Frequently Reported Oral Formulas in Randomised Controlled Trials for Shoulder-hand Syndrome

Most Common Formulas	No. of Studies	Ingredients
Bu yang huan wu tang 补阳还五汤	4 (H21, H22, H24, H25)	*Huang qi* 黄芪, *dang gui* 当归, *tao ren* 桃仁, *hong hua* 红花, *chi shao* 赤芍, *chuan xiong* 川芎 and *di long* 地龙
Huang qi gui zhi wu wu tang 黄芪桂枝五物汤	2 (H32, H37)	*Huang qi* 黄芪, *gui zhi* 桂枝, *shao yao* 芍药, *sheng jiang* 生姜 and *da zao* 大枣

Ingredients are referenced to the *Zhong Yi Fang Ji Da Ci Dian* 中医方剂大辞典 where available, or to the included study if not available.

gender, the total participants had more males (*n* = 819) than females (*n* = 534). All included studies compared the combination of oral CHM with some form of rehabilitation therapy to the same rehabilitation therapy. Four studies also utilised pharmacotherapy integrated with CHM, one study (H32) using the tropic drug piracetam in 78 people, two studies (H22, H34) using ibuprofen in 152 people, with one of these (H34) also administering vitamin B1 and the remaining study (H26) adding diclofenac in 71 people. The treatment duration of all studies varied from ten days (H54, H56, H61) to eight weeks (H26).

Only one study (H28) reported a target syndrome, utilising the CHM formula *Yi shen jie jing tang* 益肾解痉汤 for Blood stasis syndrome. Only two formulas had been evaluated by multiple studies; they are *Bu yang huan wu tang* 补阳还五汤 and *Huang qi gui zhi wu wu tang* 黄芪桂枝五物汤. See Table 5.8 for the most common formulas and Table 5.9 for the most common herbs.

Risk of Bias

Fifteen of the RCTs did not report sufficient information to rate risk of bias for sequence generation, whilst the other three studies (H28, H32, H36) were rated 'low' risk of bias as they reported using random number tables. None of the RCTs reported sufficient information to rate their risk of bias for allocation concealment. The risk of bias for blinding

Table 5.9   Frequently Reported Orally Used Herbs in Randomised Controlled Trials for Shoulder-hand Syndrome

Most Common Herbs	Scientific Name	No. of Studies
Bai shao 白芍	*Paeonia lactiflora* Pall.	11
Hong hua 红花	*Carthamus tinctorius* L.	11
Chi shao 赤芍	*Paeonia lactiflora* Pall/*Paeonia veitchii* Lynch	10
Huang qi 黄芪	*Astragalus membranaceus* (Fisch.) Bge. var. *mongholicus* (Bge.) Hsiao/*Astragalus membranaceus* (Fisch.) Bge.	9
Gui zhi 桂枝	*Cinnamomum cassia* Presl	9
Di long 地龙	*Pheretima aspergillum* (E. Perrier)/*Pheretima vulgaris* Chen/ *Pheretima guillelmi* (Michaelsen)	8
Chuan xiong 川芎	*Ligusticum chuangxiong* Hort.	7
Dang gui 当归	*Angelica sinensis* (Oliv.) Diels	7
Qiang huo 羌活	*Notopterygium* incisum Ting ex H. T. Chang/ *Notopterygium franchetii* H. de Boiss.	7
Tao ren 桃仁	*Prunus persica* (L.) Batsch/*Prunus davidiana* (Carr.) Franch.	7
Bai zhu 白术	*Atractylodes macrocephala* Koidz.	6
Fu ling 茯苓	*Poria cocos* (Schw.) Wolf	6
Gan cao 甘草	*Glycyrrhiza uralensis* Fisch./*Glycyrrhiza inflata* Bat/ *Glycyrrhiza glabra* L.	5
Dan nan xing 胆南星	*Arisaema erubescens* (Wall.) Schott/*Arisaema heterophyllum* Bl./*Arisaema amurense* Maxim.	4
Du huo 独活	*Angelica pubescens* Maxim. f. biserrata Shan et Yuan	4

of participants and personnel was rated 'high' for all studies as no blinding methods were reported. There was insufficient information reported to evaluate if outcome assessors were blinded, so the risk of bias was rated 'unclear'. None of the studies had incomplete data sets so were all rated 'low' risk for this criterion. All the studies were rated 'unclear' risk for selective outcome reporting as they did not report publication of their protocol or pre-trial registration. It was noted that one of the studies (H22) reported additional outcome measures to what was provided in the methods section, but it was evaluated that this did not raise the risk of bias in the results. Details are shown in Table 5.10.

Table 5.10   Risk of Bias of Randomised Controlled Trials: Oral Chinese Herbal Medicine for Shoulder-hand Syndrome

Risk of Bias Domain	Low Risk n (%)	Unclear Risk n (%)	High Risk n (%)
Sequence generation	3 (17.6)	14 (82.4)	0
Allocation concealment	0	17 (100)	0
Blinding of participants	0	0	17 (100)
Blinding of personnel	0	0	17
Blinding of outcome assessors	0	17 (100)	0
Incomplete outcome data	17 (100)	0	0
Selective outcome reporting	0	17 (100)	0

Outcomes for Shoulder-hand Syndrome

Of the three oral CHM RCTs which used pharmacotherapy plus rehabilitation therapy as the comparison, only one study (H34) reported FMA, ADL (BI) and pain VAS outcome. One study (H22) reported FMA and another study (H26) reported ADL (BI).

Three outcome measures were used by the included studies which compared integration of oral CHM with some form of rehabilitation therapy to the same rehabilitation therapy: 11 studies (H21, H23, H24, H27–H32, H35, H36) reported pain VAS, nine studies (H20, H24, H27–H32, H35) reported FMA and three studies (H20, H28, H32) reported ADL assessed by MBI or BI. Only two studies (H28, H32) reported all three outcome measures.

Effects of Oral Chinese Herbal Medicine for Shoulder-hand Syndrome

The effects of oral CHM for treating SHS are presented below under each outcome measure. Table 5.11 summarises the overall meta-analyses results.

Fugl-Meyer Assessment

Two studies (H26, H34) of 152 people with FMA as an outcome utilised oral CHM along with rehabilitation compared to a control

Table 5.11 Oral Chinese Herbal Medicine as Integrative Medicine: Shoulder-hand Syndrome

Comparator	Outcome	No. of Studies	No. of Participants	Effect Size (MD [95% CI])	I² %	Included Studies
Rehabilitation therapy alone	FMA	9	757	7.17 [5.46, 8.87]*	6	H20, H24, H27–H32, H35
	ADL (MBI or BI)	3	198	4.73 [1.81, 7.64]*	0	H20, H28, H32
	Pain VAS	11	871	–1.71 [–2.50, –0.91]*	95	H21, H23, H24, H27–H32, H35, H36
Pharmacotherapy plus rehabilitation	FMA	2	152	13.90 [11.45, 16.36]*	0	H26, H34
	ADL (BI)	2	129	12.34 [10.27, 14.41]*	48	H26, H34
	Pain VAS	2	152	–0.97 [–2.56, 0.61]	89	H22, H34

*Statistically significant. Abbreviations: ADL, activities of daily living; BI, Barthel Index; CI, confidence interval; FMA, Fugl-Meyer Assessment; MBI, Modified Bathel Index; MD, mean difference; VAS, visual analogue scale.

group receiving the same rehabilitation therapy as well as pharmacotherapy. Pooled results significantly favoured the CHM group (MD: 13.90 [11.45, 16.36], I² = 0%).

Nine studies (H20, H24, H27–H32, H35) of 757 people integrated oral CHM with rehabilitation therapy compared to rehabilitation therapy alone. The results from the pooled meta-analysis favoured integration of CHM compared to the rehabilitation alone for SHS using FMA as the outcome (MD: 7.17 [5.46, 8.87], I² = 6%).

Pain Score or Visual Analogue Scale

Two studies (H22, H34) of 152 people used pain VAS as an outcome. The studies integrated oral CHM with rehabilitation whilst comparing it to drugs and rehabilitation therapy. Their pooled results did not indicate statistical significant differences for pain VAS (MD: –0.97 [–2.56, 0.61], I² = 89%).

Another 11 studies (H21, H23, H24, H27–H32, H35, H36) of 871 people utilised pain VAS outcome, whilst integrating oral CHM with rehabilitation therapy compared to rehabilitation alone. The pooled results showed integrating oral CHM had greater effect (MD: –1.71 [–2.50, –0.91]); however, the heterogeneity for the group was high (I^2 = 89%).

Activities of Daily Living

Two studies (H26, H34) investigated oral CHM and rehabilitation compared to rehabilitation and pharmacotherapy in 129 people. The pooled results of BI favoured the CHM group compared to the pharmacotherapy group (MD: 11.27 [6.56, 15.98], I^2 = 48%).

Another three studies (H20, H28, H32) of 198 people integrated oral CHM with rehabilitation compared to rehabilitation alone. Pooled results indicated improvement in ADL (MBI or BI) favoured the oral CHM group (MD: 4.73 [1.81, 7.64], I^2 = 0%).

Randomised Controlled Trial Evidence for Individual Oral Formulas: Shoulder-hand Syndrome

Of the studies utilising the same CHM formula, FMA was reported for two studies (H20, H29) using *Zi ni bu qi hua tan tong luo fang* 自拟补气化痰通络方. When pooled, the results favoured the combination of oral CHM and rehabilitation therapy (MD: 4.14 [0.80, 7.48], I^2 = 0%).

Two studies (H21, H24) using the formula of *Bu yang huan wu tang* 补阳还五汤 and two studies (H30, H31) using *Zi ni tong luo huo xue tang* 自拟通络活血汤 reported pain VAS as an outcome. Meta-analysis of the two studies using *Zi ni tong luo huo xue tang* 自拟通络活血汤 showed it had a significant improvement in pain VAS compared to the control group (MD: –1.35 [–1.89, –0.82], I^2 = 0%) (H30, H31). For *Bu yang huan wu tang* 补阳还五汤, a meta-analysis of the two studies showed overall there was no statistical significant difference for pain VAS with the control group (MD: –2.91 [–7.03, 1.22], I^2 = 99%) (H21, H24).

The two studies (H32, H37) utilising *Huang qi gui zhi wu wu tang* 黄芪桂枝五物汤 were not pooled in the meta-analysis, as one study (H37) utilised both oral and topical CHM interventions.

Frequently Reported Orally Used Herbs in Meta-analyses Showing Favourable Effect for Shoulder-hand Syndrome

The most frequent herbs used in studies from favourable meta-analyses were calculated (Table 5.12). Studies were grouped according to the outcome measures (FMA, ADL or pain VAS) regardless of their comparator (rehabilitation therapy alone or with pharmacotherapy).

Non-controlled Studies of Oral Chinese Herbal Medicine

Two non-controlled studies of 58 people utilised oral CHM, with neither study reporting their target syndrome. One study (H38) used oral *Yi shen juan bi tang* 益肾蠲痹汤 in 26 people (containing: *Dang gui* 当归, *di huang* 地黄, *yan hu suo* 延胡索, wu *shao she* 乌梢蛇, *quan xie* 全蝎, *yin yang huo* 淫羊藿, *gu sui bu* 骨碎补, *di long* 地龙, *lou feng fang* 露蜂房 and *tu bie chong* 土鳖虫). The other study of 32 people (H39) did not state the formula name, but did detail the ingredients (*huang qi* 黄芪, *chi shao* 赤芍, *chuanxiong* 川芎, *dang gui* 当归, *di long* 地龙, *hong hua* 红花, *tao ren* 桃仁, *niu xi* 牛膝, *sang ji sheng* 桑寄生, *gui zhi* 桂枝, *ru xiang* 乳香, *mo yao* 没药, *fu ling* 茯苓, *ze xie* 泽泻, *gan cao* 甘草 and *quan xie* 全蝎). Both studies utilised effective rate as an outcome, with only one of the studies (H39) reporting FMA and neither study reporting adverse events.

Topical Chinese Herbal Medicine for Shoulder-hand Syndrome

Topical CHM was the most frequent form of administration in studies for SHS, with 34 RCTs, one non-randomised controlled trial and six non-controlled studies.

Table 5.12 Frequently Reported Orally Used Herbs in Meta-analyses Showing Favourable Effect for Shoulder-hand Syndrome

Outcome Measure	No. of Meta-analyses	No. of Studies	Herbs	Scientific Name	No. of Studies Using Herb
FMA	2	11	*Di long* 地龙	*Pheretima aspergillum* (E. Perrier)/ *Pheretima vulgaris* Chen/*Pheretima guillelmi* (Michaelsen)	7
			Bai shao 白芍	*Paeonia lactiflora* Pall.	4
			Chuan xiong 川芎	*Ligusticum chuangxiong* Hort.	4
			Gan cao 甘草	*Glycyrrhiza uralensis* Fisch./ *Glycyrrhiza inflata* Bat./ *Glycyrrhiza glabra* L.	4
			Chi shao 赤芍	*Paeonia lactiflora* Pall./*Paeonia veitchii* Lynch	3
			Dang gui 当归	Angelica sinensis (Oliv.) Diels	3
			Tao ren 桃仁	*Prunus persica* (L.) Batsch/*Prunus davidiana* (Carr.) Franch.	3
			Gui zhi 桂枝	*Cinnamomum cassia* Presl	3
			Hong hua 红花	*Carthamus tinctorius* L.	3
			Qiang huo 羌活	*Notopterygium* incisum Ting ex H. T. Chang/ *Notopterygium franchetii* H. de Boiss.	3
			Sang zhi 桑枝	*Morus alba* L.	3
ADL	2	5	*Di long* 地龙	*Pheretima aspergillum* (E. Perrier) / *Pheretima vulgaris* Chen/ *Pheretima guillelmi* (Michaelsen)	4
			Chuan xiong 川芎	*Ligusticum chuangxiong* Hort.	2
			Dang gui 当归	Angelica sinensis (Oliv.) Diels	2
			Gui zhi 桂枝	*Cinnamomum cassia* Presl	2
			Sang zhi 桑枝	*Morus alba* L.	2
			Bai shao 白芍	*Paeonia lactiflora* Pall.	2
			Ji xue teng 鸡血藤	*Spatholobus suberectus* Dunn	2
Pain VAS	1	11	*Di long* 地龙	*Pheretima aspergillum* (E. Perrier) / *Pheretima vulgaris* Chen/ *Pheretima guillelmi* (Michaelsen)	5
			Chuan xiong 川芎	*Ligusticum chuangxiong* Hort.	5

(Continued)

Table 5.12   (*Continued*)

Outcome Measure	No. of Meta-analyses	No. of Studies	Herbs	Scientific Name	No. of Studies Using Herb
			Chi shao 赤芍	*Paeonia lactiflora* Pall./*Paeonia veitchii* Lynch	5
			Bai shao 白芍	*Paeonia lactiflora* Pall.	5
			Tao ren 桃仁	*Prunus persica* (L.) Batsch/*Prunus davidiana* (Carr.) Franch.	4
			Hong hua 红花	*Carthamus tinctorius* L.	4
			Gan cao 甘草	*Glycyrrhiza uralensis* Fisch./ *Glycyrrhiza inflata* Bat./ *Glycyrrhiza glabra* L.	4
			Qiang huo 羌活	*Notopterygium* incisum Ting ex H. T. Chang/*Notopterygium franchetii* H. de Boiss.	4
			Gui zhi 桂枝	*Cinnamomum cassia* Presl	3
			Fu ling 茯苓	*Poria cocos* (Schw.) Wolf	3

Abbreviations: ADL, activities of daily living; FMA, Fugl-Meyer Assessment; VAS, visual analogue scale.

Randomised Controlled Trials of Topical Chinese Herbal Medicine

A total of 34 RCTs (H40–H73) investigated topical CHM for SHS in 2,300 subjects. For those studies that reported the participant gender, there were more males ($n = 569$) than females ($n = 413$). All studies combined a topical CHM with some form of rehabilitation therapy with a treatment duration ranging from ten days in three studies (H54, H61, H62) to one month in nine studies (H46, H48–H50, H60, H62, H65, H68, H69).

CHM bath therapy was utilised as the CHM administration form by 11 studies (H42–H44, H47–H49, H51, H53–H55, H73) totaling 877 people compared to rehabilitation therapy. Eleven studies (H46, H50, H56–H59, H68–H72) utilised CHM fomentation combined with rehabilitation compared to rehabilitation alone. Ten studies (H45, H52, H60–H67) used CHM steam therapy in 627 people, all comparing the combination of CHM and rehabilitation to rehabilitation alone, with two studies also using nerve block therapy (H60) or warm water therapy (H61). In addition, two studies (H40, H41) of 90 people combined the external application of CHM to rehabilitation and compared it to rehabilitation alone.

None of the studies reported the use of syndrome differentiation. Ten studies (H40, H41, H46–H48, H50, H55, H67, H71, H72). reported the name of their CHM topical formulas. None of these studies though utilised the same CHM formula. Frequently used herbs are listed in Table 5.13.

Risk of Bias

Of the 34 RCTs, eight (H42, H52–H55, H62, H70, H71) were rated 'low' risk of bias for sequence generation as they utilised random number tables. The remaining 28 RCTs were rated 'unclear' risk as they did not report their sequence generation methods. All the RCTs were rated 'unclear' risk for allocation concealment as they did not report sufficient information to make a clear judgment. All the RCTs were rated 'high' risk for blinding of participants and personnel as the studies did not report utilising placebos. The blinding of outcome assessors was rated 'unclear' risk for all RCTs as the reported information was insufficient to make clear judgement. All the RCTs were rated 'low' risk for incomplete outcome data as they appeared to report all participant outcome results. It was noted that one of the RCTs (H50) did report one drop out; however, it was judged unlikely to significantly bias the study. For selective outcome reporting, four of the included RCTs (H41, H50, H55, H64) were rated 'high' risk of bias for selective outcome reporting. All four studies reported collecting outcome data in their methods section which were not provided in the results sections. Details are shown in Table 5.14.

Outcomes for Shoulder-hand Syndrome

The 34 integrated topical CHM and rehabilitation therapy studies evaluated four outcome measures for shoulder-hand syndrome. Similar

Table 5.13   Frequently Reported Topically Used Herbs in Randomised Controlled Trials for Shoulder-hand Syndrome

Most Common Herbs	Scientific Name	No. of Studies
Hong hua 红花	*Carthamus tinctorius* L.	28
Tou gu cao 透骨草	Herba Clematidis Intricatae	19
Shen jin cao 伸筋草	*Lycopodium japonicum* Thunb.	18
Gui zhi 桂枝	*Cinnamomum cassia* Presl	18
Dang gui 当归	*Angelica sinensis* Oliv. Diels	16
Chuan xiong 川芎	*Ligusticum chuangxiong* Hort.	14
Ru xiang 乳香	*Boswellia carterii* Birdw./*Boswellia bhaw-dajiana* Birdw.	13
Mo yao 没药	*Commiphora myrrha* Engl./*Commiphora molmol* Engl.	12
Sang zhi 桑枝	*Morus alba* L.	12
Wei ling xian 威灵仙	*Clematis chinensis* Osbeck/*Clematis hexapetala* Pall./*Clematis manshurica* Rupr.	13
Tao ren 桃仁	*Prunus persica* L. Batsch/*Prunus davidiana* Carr. Franch.	9
Ji xue teng 鸡血藤	*Spatholobus suberectus* Dunn	8
Fang feng 蜂房	*Polistes olivaceous* DeGeer/*Polistes japonicus* Saussure/*Parapolybia varia* Fabricius	7
Du huo 独活	*Angelica pubescens* Maxim. f. *biserrata* Shan et Yuan	7
Bai shao 白芍	*Paeonia lactiflora* Pall.	6
Mu gua 木瓜	*Chaenomeles speciosa* Sweet Nakai	6
Niu xi 牛膝	*Achyranthes bidentata* Bl.	6

to the oral CHM studies, FMA, ADL and pain VAS were investigated with the addition of the numerical rating scale (NRS). No study reported all outcome measures. Fourteen studies (H41, H42, H47, H49, H52–H54, H60, H62, H64–H66, H69, H71) investigated FMA and 14 studies (H40, H41, H43, H47, H53, H54, H57, H60, H62, H64–H66, H70, H72) reported data on pain VAS, whilst only four studies (H41, H49, H59, H71) reported data on ADL and three studies (H42, H55,

Table 5.14   Risk of Bias of Randomised Controlled Trials: Topical Chinese Herbal Medicine for Shoulder-hand Syndrome

Risk of Bias Domain	Low Risk n (%)	Unclear Risk n (%)	High Risk n (%)
Sequence generation	6 (17.6)	28 (82.3)	0
Allocation concealment	0	34	0
Blinding of participants	0	0	34 (100)
Blinding of personnel	0	0	34 (100)
Blinding of outcome assessors	0	34 (100)	0
Incomplete outcome data	34 (100)	0	0
Selective outcome reporting	0	30 (88.2)	4 (11.8)

H71) for NRS scale. One study (H54) did not report end-of-treatment effects and another (H73) included additional interventions that were not in the control group so the true effect of CHM was unknown. Both these studies were excluded from the meta-analysis.

Two studies (H46, H48) utilised a topical CHM compared to cold and hot water therapy in which FMA was the only outcome reported; however, they did not report their end-of-treatment data to enable analysis.

Subgroup analyses were performed with studies pooled according to their CHM form of application: CHM steam therapy, bath, fomentation or external application.

Effects of Topical Chinese Herbal Medicine for Shoulder-hand Syndrome

The effects of topical CHM for treating SHS are presented below under each outcome measures. Table 5.15 summarises the overall meta-analysis results and Table 5.16 lists the subgroup meta-analysis results.

Fugl-Meyer Assessment

Thirteen (H41, H42, H47, H49, H52, H53, H60, H62, H64–H66, H69, H71) topical CHM studies of 865 people were poolable using

Table 5.15 Topical Chinese Herbal Medicine as Integrative Medicine vs. Rehabilitation Therapy: Shoulder-hand Syndrome

Outcome	No. of Studies	No. of Participants	Effect Size (MD [95% CI])	I² %	Included Studies
FMA	13	865	7.27 [3.57, 10.97]*	98	H41, H42, H47, H49, H52, H53, H60, H62, H64–H66, H69, H71
ADL (MBI or BI)	4	234	12.75 [7.16, 18.33]*	94	H41, H49, H59, H71
Pain VAS	13	821	−1.92 [−2.31, −1.53]*	88	H40, H41, H43, H47, H53, H52, H60, H62, H64–H66, H70, H72
NRS	3	253	−1.25 [−1.91, −0.59]*	76	H42, H55, H71

*Statistically significant. Abbreviations: ADL, activities of daily living; BI, Barthel Index; CI, confidence interval; FMA, Fugl-Meyer Assessment; MBI, Modified Barthel Index; MD, mean difference; NRS, numerical rating scale; VAS, visual analogue scale.

Table 5.16 Topical Chinese Herbal Medicine as Integrative Medicine for Shoulder-hand Syndrome Subgroup Analyses

Intervention	Outcome	No. of Studies	No. of Participants	Effect Size (MD [95% CI])	I² %	Included Studies
CHM steam therapy	FMA	6	367	7.48 [1.32, 13.64]*	96	H52, H60, H62, H64–H66
	Pain VAS	4	247	−1.82 [−2.40, −1.24]*	80	H60, H62, H65, H66
Fomentation	FMA	2	114	4.55 [0.43, 8.67]*	95	H69, H70
	ADL (MBI or BI)	2	103	9.01 [6.67, 11.36]*	33	H59, H71
	Pain VAS	3	180	−3.40 [−5.51, −1.29]*	91	H57, H70, H72
CHM bath therapy	FMA	4	324	7.16 [−2.78, 17.11]	99	H42, H47, H49, H53
	Pain VAS	4	304	−1.37 [−1.60, −1.15]*	16	H43, H47, H52, H53
	NRS	2	153	−1.33 [−2.44, −0.22]*	88	H42, H55
	Pain VAS	2	90	−1.73 [−3.01, −0.45]*	91	H40, H41

*Statistically significant. Abbreviations: ADL, activities of daily living; BI, Barthel Index; CI, confidence interval; FMA, Fugl-Meyer Assessment; MBI, Modified Barthel Index; MD, mean difference; NRS, numerical rating scale; VAS, visual analogue scale.

the outcome FMA. The results of the meta-analysis favoured application of CHM and rehabilitation, compared to rehabilitation therapy alone (MD: 7.27 [3.57, 10.97], I^2 = 98%). The high heterogeneity was likely due to variation between the topical administration forms for each study so further subgroup analysis was conducted based on CHM treatment form.

Subgroup analysis favoured the integration of CHM steam therapy (MD: 7.48 [1.32, 13.64], I^2 = 96%) (H52, H60, H62, H64–H66) and CHM fomentation (MD: 4.55 [0.43, 8.67], I^2 = 95%) (H69, H71). However, integrating CHM bath therapy with rehabilitation did not improve FMA outcome effects (MD: 7.16 [–2.78, 17.11], I^2 = 99%). There was high heterogeneity for each of these subgroups which may be due to variation in measuring the FMA outcome or variation in design of the studies. For the studies using CHM steam therapy, when a sensitivity analysis was conducted based on treatment duration, removing two studies that applied treatment for less than four weeks duration (H52, H62) saw the overall effect further increase (MD: 8.23 [5.57, 10.88]) and heterogeneity reduce (I^2 = 40%). A sensitivity analysis of the bath therapy subgroup was unable to explain the heterogeneity as the durations of treatment were similar for all the studies. However, two studies (H47, H49) did not report the duration of the condition, which if they did differ significantly from the other studies, may have impacted the treatment effects. Similarly, one of the two studies in the fomentation subgroup (H69) did not report duration of condition which might explain their heterogeneity.

The FMA outcome was reported by only one study using the external application of CHM (H41), and favoured its use along with rehabilitation (MD: 12.98 [10.10, 15.86]).

Further, two studies with FMA as the outcome combined topical CHM with rehabilitation therapy and compared it to the same rehabilitation therapy combined with cold/hot water therapy. One of these studies (H46) utilised CHM in fomentation form with 48 participants and the other (H48) as bath therapy with 42 participants. Neither of the studies reported end-of-treatment FMA outcome data so they could not be pooled in meta-analysis.

Pain: Numerical Ratings Score or Visual Analogue Scale

Thirteen studies reported poolable pain VAS scores in 821 people. The results indicated that integrating topical CHM with rehabilitation was more effective for pain VAS than without CHM (MD: −1.92 [−2.31, −1.53], I^2 = 88%). The high heterogeneity of the studies was explored using subgroup analysis, again according to the form of administration. All subgroups showed they favoured integration of CHM and rehabilitation to improve pain VAS, with four studies (H60, H62, H65, H66) investigating CHM steam therapy (MD: −1.82 [−2.40, −1.24], I^2 = 80%), three studies (H57, H70, H72) of CHM fomentation (MD: −3.40 [−5.51, −1.29], I^2 = 91%), four studies (H43, H47, H53, H64) of CHM bath therapy (MD: −1.37 [−1.60, −1.15], I^2 = 16%) and two studies (H40, H41) of CHM external application (MD: −1.73 [−3.01, −0.45], I^2 = 91%). The heterogeneity was low for the bath therapy subgroup of studies; however, for the other subgroups it was high.

For the CHM steam therapy group, a sensitivity analysis was conducted based on treatment duration. One study (H62) was removed as it applied treatment for less than four weeks. Results still favoured integrating CHM, yet showed no heterogeneity (MD: −2.16 [−2.40, −1.93], I^2 = 0%). Treatment durations were similar amongst the CHM fomentation studies; however, disease duration had significant difference between two of the studies (H57, H72), and the third (H70) did not report disease duration; this may explain their heterogeneity. The two studies (H40, H41) using CHM external application of CHM applied treatment for similar durations and participants had similar disease duration, so the reason for high heterogeneity was unclear.

Activities of Daily Living

Four studies (H41, H49, H59, H71) reported ADL using BI or MBI as an outcome poolable for SHS in 234 people. Meta-analysis indicated their effect favoured administering topical CHM along with rehabilitation therapy (MD: 12.75 [7.16, 18.33], I^2 = 94%), although with high heterogeneity. Subgrouping the studies in the meta-analysis was only possible for two studies (H59, H71) which both used CHM fomentation and favoured its application (MD: 9.01 [6.67, 11.36] $I^2 = 33\%$). For the other two studies, one (H49) utilised CHM bath therapy (MD: 19.90 [16.97, 22.83]) and the other (H41) CHM external application (MD: 14.60 [11.05, 18.15]).

Effective Rate

Twenty-five RCTs utilised some form of effective rate as an outcome in 1,730 people; however, as there was variation in how the effective rate was determined, they were not pooled in the meta-analysis.

Assessment Using GRADE

Through the consensus process, it was determined that a summary of findings table should be prepared for the comparison of topical CHM combined with routine rehabilitation vs. rehabilitation alone. Thirteen studies (H41, H42, H47, H49, H52, H53, H60, H62, H64–H66, H69, H71) reported data on FMA, four studies (H41, H49, H59, H71) reported ADL and 13 studies (H40, H41, H43, H47, H53, H52, H60, H62, H64–H66, H70, H72) reported pain score or VAS. Evidence for topical CHM as integrative medicine with routine rehabilitation for these three outcomes is "low" or "very low" certainty, although significant benefit of adding topical CHM was found in all meta-analyses or subgroup meta-analyses (Table 5.17).

Randomised Controlled Trial Evidence for Individual Topical Formulas

No study reported using the same formulas as well as reporting the same outcome measure data for meta-analysis. Of the named formulas, none of them directly corresponded to formulas from Chapter 2.

Frequently Reported Topically Used Herbs in Meta-analyses Showing Favourable Effect for Shoulder-hand Syndrome

The most frequently reported herbs from studies favouring integration of topical CHM with rehabilitation for SHS were calculated

Table 5.17 GRADE: Topical Chinese Herbal Medicine Plus Routine Rehabilitation Compared to Routine Rehabilitation for Post-stroke Shoulder-hand Syndrome

Outcomes	No. of Participants (Studies) Follow-up	Certainty of the Evidence (GRADE)	Anticipated Absolute Effects	
			Risk with Rehabilitation	Risk Difference with Topical CHM + Rehabilitation
FMA	865 (13 RCTs)	⊕⊕◯◯ LOW[a,b]	The mean FMA was **29.95**	MD **7.27 higher** (3.57 higher to 10.97 higher)
FMA — steam	367 (6 RCTs)	⊕◯◯◯ VERY LOW[a,b,c]	The mean FMA — steam was **26.11**	MD **7.48 higher** (1.32 higher to 13.64 higher)
FMA — bath	324 (4 RCTs)	⊕◯◯◯ VERY LOW[a,b,c]	The mean FMA — bath was **32.59**	MD **7.16 higher** (2.78 lower to 17.11 higher)
FMA — fomentation	114 (2 RCTs)	⊕◯◯◯ VERY LOW[a,b,c]	The mean FMA — fomentation was **27.30**	MD **4.55 higher** (0.43 higher to 8.67 higher)
FMA — external application	60 (1 RCT)	⊕⊕◯◯ LOW[a,c]	The mean FMA — external application was **44.1**	MD **12.98 higher** (10.1 higher to 15.86 higher)
ADL	234 (4 RCTs)	⊕◯◯◯ VERY LOW[a,b,c]	The mean ADL was **60.73**	MD **12.75 higher** (7.16 higher to 18.33 higher)
ADL — fomentation	103 (2 RCTs)	⊕⊕◯◯ LOW[a,c]	The mean ADL — fomentation was **61.52**	MD **9.01 higher** (6.67 higher to 11.36 higher)
ADL — bath	71 (1 RCT)	⊕⊕◯◯ LOW[a,c]	The mean ADL — bath was **66.5**	MD **19.9 higher** (16.97 higher to 22.83 higher)
ADL — external application	60 (1 RCT)	⊕⊕◯◯ LOW[a,c]	The mean ADL — external application was **51.75**	MD **14.6 higher** (11.05 higher to 18.15 higher)

(Continued)

Table 5.17 (*Continued*)

Outcomes	No. of Participants (Studies) Follow-up	Certainty of the Evidence (GRADE)	Anticipated Absolute Effects	
			Risk with Rehabilitation	Risk Difference with Topical CHM + Rehabilitation
Pain VAS	821 (13 RCTs)	⊕⊕◯◯ LOW[a,b]	The mean VAS was **4.49**	MD **1.92 lower** (2.31 lower to 1.53 lower)
Pain VAS — steam	247 (4 RCTs)	⊕◯◯◯ VERY LOW[a,b,c]	The mean VAS — steam was **4.33**	MD **1.82 lower** (2.4 lower to 1.24 lower)
Pain VAS — fomentation	180 (3 RCTs)	⊕◯◯◯ VERY LOW[a,b,c]	The mean VAS — fomentation was **6.59**	MD **3.4 lower** (5.51 lower to 1.29 lower)
Pain VAS — bath	304 (4 RCTs)	⊕⊕◯◯ LOW[a,c]	The mean VAS — bath was **3.43**	MD **1.37 lower** (1.6 lower to 1.15 lower)
Pain VAS — external application	90 (2 RCTs)	⊕◯◯◯ VERY LOW[a,b,c]	The mean VAS — external application was **4.29**	MD **1.73 lower** (3.01 lower to 0.45 lower)
Adverse events	(1 RCT)		The study reported there was no adverse event observed.	

The risk in the intervention group (and its 95% confidence interval) is based on the assumed risk in the comparison group and the relative effect of the intervention (and its 95% CI).

Abbreviations: ADL, activities of daily living; CHM, Chinese herbal medicine; CI, confidence interval; FMA, Fugl-Meyer Assessment; GRADE, Grading of Recommendations Assessment, Development and Evaluation; MD, mean difference; RCT, randomised control trial; VAS, visual analogue scale.

Notes:

a. Lack of blinding of participants and personnel.
b. Substantial statistical heterogeneity.
c. Small sample size limits certainty of results.

Study References:

FMA: H41, H42, H47, H49, H52, H53, H60, H62, H64–H66, H69, H71
FMA — steam: H52, H60, H62, H64–H66
FMA — bath: H42, H47, H49, H53
FMA — fomentation: H69, H70
FMA — external application: H41
ADL: H41, H49, H59, H71
ADL — fomentation: H59, H71
ADL — bath: H49
ADL — external application: H41
Pain VAS: H40, H41, H43, H47, H53, H52, H60, H62, H64–H66, H70, H72
Pain VAS — steam: H60, H62, H65, H66
Pain VAS — fomentation: H57, H70, H72
Pain VAS — bath: H43, H47, H52, H53
Pain VAS — external application: H40, H41

Adverse events: H53

and are presented in Table 5.18. Frequency is grouped according to the form of CHM intervention (steam therapy or fomentation) and the meta-analysis SHS outcome measure (FMA, ADL, pain VAS or NRS). Only two external application studies (H40, H41) were pooled with a favourable meta-analysis outcome for pain VAS, so frequency for these studies was calculated. Topical CHM bath therapy studies did not show a favourable result when pooled in the meta-analysis so herb frequency of these studies is not shown in Table 5.18.

Controlled Clinical Trials (Non-randomised) of Topical Chinese Herbal Medicine

Only one CCT (H74) utilised topical CHM for SHS. The study did not report the name of the formula or the treating syndrome; it did, however, provide the ingredients which were administered. These were administered as bath therapy for ten days, 45 minutes at a time (CHM ingredients: *hong hua* 红花, *cao wu* 草乌, *chuan wu* 川乌, *dang gui* 当归, *chuan xiong* 川芎, *sang zhi* 桑枝, *gui zhi* 桂枝). This study reported the change scores of pain VAS, FMA and ADL; there was no between-group difference in terms of these outcomes. However, the sample size of this study is quite small (20 vs. 10 participants).

Non-controlled Studies of Topical Chinese Herbal Medicine

A total of six (H75–H80) non-controlled studies utilised topical CHM for SHS in 245 people and all integrated some form of movement therapy with no adverse events reported. Two of the studies (H75, H80) also administered electrical stimulation therapy.

Three studies (H76, H77, H79) administered CHM steam therapy in 137 people, two studies (H75, H78) in 70 people as CHM bath therapy and one study (H80) in 38 people as externally applied CHM. Only two studies reported the name of the formulas they used for external application: one using *Shu jing huo luo xi ji* 舒筋活络洗剂)

Table 5.18   Frequently Reported Topically Used Herbs from the Meta-analyses Showing Favourable Effect for Shoulder-hand Syndrome: Fomentation, Steam Therapy and Bath Therapy

Outcome Measure	No. of Meta-analyses	No. of Studies	Herbs	Scientific Name	No. of Studies Using Herb
FMA	1	13	Hong hua 红花	*Carthamus tinctorius* L.	8
			Shen jin cao 伸筋草	*Lycopodium japonicum* Thunb.	5
			Dang gui 当归	*Angelica sinensis* Oliv. Diels	5
			Gui zhi 桂枝	*Cinnamomum cassia* Presl	5
			Sang zhi 桑枝	*Morus alba* L.	5
			Ru xiang 乳香	*Boswellia carterii* Birdw./ *Boswellia bhaw-dajiana* Birdw.	5
			Mo yao 没药	*Commiphora myrrha* Engl./ *Commiphora molmol* Engl	4
			Tou gu cao 透骨草	Herba Clematidis Intricatae	4
			Chuan xiong 川芎	*Ligusticum chuangxiong* Hort.	4
			Di long 地龙	*Pheretima aspergillum* E. Perrier/ *Pheretima vulgaris* Chen/ *Pheretima guillelmi* Michaelsen	4
ADL	1	4	Hong hua 红花	*Carthamus tinctorius* L.	2
Pain VAS or NRS	2		Hong hua 红花	*Carthamus tinctorius* L.	10
			Ru xiang 乳香	*Boswellia carterii* Birdw./ *Boswellia bhaw-dajiana* Birdw.	7
			Mo yao 没药	*Commiphora myrrha* Engl./ *Commiphora molmol* Engl	7
			Gui zhi 桂枝	*Cinnamomum cassia* Presl	6
			Sang zhi 桑枝	*Morus alba* L.	6
			Shen jin cao 伸筋草	*Lycopodium japonicum* Thunb.	5
			Tou gu cao 透骨草	Herba Clematidis Intricatae	5
			Di long 地龙	*Pheretima aspergillum* E. Perrier/ *Pheretima vulgaris* Chen/ *Pheretima guillelmi* Michaelsen	5
			Dang gui 当归	*Angelica sinensis* Oliv. Diels	5
			Huang qi 黄芪	*Astragalus membranaceus* Fisch. Bge. var. *mongholicus* Bge. Hsiao/ *Astragalus membranaceus* Fisch. Bge.	5

Abbreviations: ADL, activities of daily living; FMA, Fugl-Meyer Assessment; VAS, visual analogue scale.

Table 5.19 Frequently Reported Topically Used Herbs in Non-controlled Studies

Most Common Herbs	Scientific Name	No. of Studies
Gui zhi 桂枝	*Cinnamomum cassia* Presl	5
Hong hua 红花	*Carthamus tinctorius* L.	4
Mo yao 没药	*Commiphora myrrha* Engl./*Commiphora molmol* Engl.	4
Xi xin 细辛	*Asarum heterotropoides* Fr. Schmidt var. *mandshuricum* (Maxim) Kitag./*Asarum sieboldii* Miq. var. *seoulense* Nakai/*Asarum sieboldii* Miq.	4
Ru xiang 乳香	*Boswellia carterii* Birdw./*Boswellia bhaw-dajiana* Birdw.	3
Tou gu cao 透骨草	*Herba Clematidis Intricatae*	3
Chuan xiong 川芎	*Ligusticum chuangxiong* Hort.	2
Dang gui 当归	*Angelica sinensis* (Oliv.) Diels	2
Di long 地龙	*Pheretima aspergillum* (E. Perrier)/*Pheretima vulgaris* Chen/*Pheretima guillelmi* (Michaelsen)/*Pheretima pectinifera* Michaelsen	2
Mu gua 木瓜	*Chaenomeles speciosa* (Sweet) Nakai	2
Shen jin cao 伸筋草	*Lycopodium japonicum* Thunb.	2

Note: The use of some herbs may be restricted in some countries. Readers are advised to comply with relevant regulations.

(H75) and the other using *Si huang shui mi* 四黄水蜜 (ingredients: *Huang qi* 黄芩, *huang lian* 黄连, *huang bai* 黄柏, *da huang* 大黄, and honey 蜜糖) (H78). One of these studies (H78) allowed for bath, in addition to the CHM external application, yet did not state the name of the CHM bath formula. Frequently used herbs are listed in Table 5.19.

A variety of outcome measures were utilised with reporting of FMA, ADL and pain VAS by one study (H75). Effective rate was reported by four studies (H76, H78–H80), whilst one study (H76) reported data on Brunstrom stages.

Oral Plus Topical Chinese Herbal Medicine for Shoulder-hand Syndrome

Only four RCTs were found investigating oral plus topical CHM.

Randomised Controlled Trials of Oral Plus Topical Chinese Herbal Medicine

Four RCTs (H37, H81–H83), consisting of 428 participants, investigated the combination of oral and topical CHM, compared to some form of conventional therapy. All studies combined CHM with rehabilitation of some type, and one study (H82) also delivered Stellate Ganglion Block therapy to both the intervention CHM ($n = 40$) and control groups ($n = 40$).

No studies reported using the same topical CHM. One study of 90 people (H37) administered one of three different oral formulas (modified *Huang qi gui zhi wu wu tang* 黄芪桂枝五味汤加减, modified *Shuang he tang* 双合汤加减 or modified *Liu wei di huang wan* 六味地黄丸加减). The administration of each CHM formula was based on each participant's syndrome and combined treatment with another unnamed CHM bath formula. This study could not be pooled with the other studies as it only reported effective rate data (H37). For the remaining three studies, only one (H83) reported the names of the CHM formula used (oral: *Xi xian tong luo fang* 豨莶通络方; topical: *Xi xian tong luo ye* 豨莶通络液). Each of the studies used a different form of topical CHM: external application (H81), fomentation (H82) and bath (H83).

One study (H82) did not report syndrome type whilst the other three studies (H37, H81, H83) reported different syndromes, although Phlegm stagnation and Blood stasis was an aspect of syndrome for the other three studies. One study reported the entire syndrome as *qi* 气 deficiency, Blood stasis, Phlegm stagnation, and Liver and Kidney deficiency (H37). Another (H81) reported syndrome as *yang qi* 阳气, deficiency combined with Phlegm stagnation and Blood stasis, while the remaining study (H83) reported syndrome as Wind invasion combined with Phlegm stagnation and Blood stasis.

Risk of Bias

Two studies (H81, H83) were rated 'low' risk of bias for sequence generation as they reported using random number tables. The other two studies (H37, H82) were rated as 'unclear' risk without sufficient details reported to make a judgment. All the RCTs were rated 'unclear' risk for allocation concealment and rated 'high' risk for blinding of participants and personnel. Blinding of outcome assessors was rated as 'unclear' risk for all four studies and assessment of incomplete outcome data was considered 'low' risk for all studies. Selective reporting bias was 'unclear' risk as none of the studies published their protocol.

Outcome for Shoulder-hand Syndrome

As mentioned, one study (H37) only reported effective rate data. For the remaining three studies, each reported FMA and pain VAS, with one of the studies (H83) also reporting ADL along with two uncommon outcome measures.

Effects of Oral Plus Topical Chinese Herbal Medicine for Shoulder-hand Syndrome

The effects of oral plus topical CHM for SHS are presented below under each outcome measures. Meta-analyses results are listed in Table 5.20.

Fugl-Meyer Assessment

Three RCTs (H81–H83) investigated combination of oral and topical CHM integrated with rehabilitation therapy in 230 people

Table 5.20   Oral Plus Topical Chinese Herbal Medicine as Integrative Medicine vs. Pharmacotherapy

Intervention	Comparator	Outcome	No. of Studies	No. of Participants	Effect Size (MD [95% CI])	I² %	Included Studies
Oral plus topical CHM as IM	Pharmacotherapy	FMA	3	230	8.39 [7.20, 9.58]*	0	H81–H83
		Pain VAS	3	230	−1.70 [−3.02, −0.39]*	98	H81–H83

*Statistically significant. Abbreviations: CHM, Chinese herbal medicine; IM: integrative medicine; CI, confidence interval; FMA, Fugl-Meyer Assessment; MD, mean difference.

using FMA as the outcome for SHS. Pooled meta-analysis showed the CHM integrated treatment to be superior to rehabilitation alone (MD: 8.39 [7.20, 9.58], $I^2 = 0\%$). Two of the studies (H81, H83) detailed syndrome information with both involving phlegm stagnation and Blood stasis.

Pain Score or Visual Analogue Scale

Three RCTs (H81–H83) reported pain VAS for SHS. The meta-analysis of their pooled effect data favoured integration of oral and topical CHM with rehabilitation therapy in SHS (MD: −1.70 [−3.02, −0.39], $I^2 = 98\%$). There was high heterogeneity for the pooled studies so a sensitivity analysis was conducted based on treatment duration. Two of the studies (H81, H83) applied treatment for approximately four weeks and the other study (H82) just two weeks. When the shorter duration study was removed, integration of CHM remained favourable; however, heterogeneity substantially reduced (MD: −1.08 [−1.37, −0.79], $I^2 = 0\%$).

Activities of Daily Living

Only one study (H83) reported ADL (MBI) outcome data, which found from 60 participants that there was no greater ADL improvement with the integration of topical and oral CHM to rehabilitation.

Effective Rate

Two studies (H37, H81) reported effective rate as the outcome in 288 people; however, they were not pooled in meta-analysis as their methods of calculation for effective rate were unclear.

Safety of Chinese Herbal Medicine

Three RCTs of oral CHM reported information of adverse events; two of these studies in 154 people (H22, H28) reported there were no such events observed. The remaining study of 71 people (H26) reported two cases of stomach upset in the control group and no adverse effects reported for the CHM group.

Two RCTs of topical CHM (H7, H53) reported the collection of adverse events data; however, they both reported no adverse events observed during the studies. There was no adverse event caused by the topical use of CHM. One RCT, utilising both oral and topical CHM (H83), reported collecting adverse events data; however, it reported that no adverse events were observed.

None of the non-controlled studies or non-randomised CCTs reported details on adverse events.

Evidence for Chinese Herbal Medicine Treatments Commonly Used in Clinical Practice

The common practice of CHM for stroke recommended by guidelines and textbooks is summarised in Chapter 2. Topical CHM has been recommended by multiple guidelines being used as a bath therapy applied on the paralytic extremities. Among the clinical studies, topical CHM has been evaluated when it was used as CHM bath therapy, CHM fomentation, CHM steam therapy and CHM external application. However, most of these studies did not provide the names of their topical CHM formulas. In terms of the orally taken CHM formulas, *Bu yang huan wu tang* 补阳还五汤 is the chief formula for post-stroke extremity complications (as summarised in Chapter 2). Consistently, this formula is also the most frequently used one in the included studies of oral CHM. However, meta-analysis of only two studies did not support the add-on benefit in terms of pain VAS of this formula.

In terms of the herb ingredients, it is noted that the herbs which have the function of moving Blood stasis, unblocking collaterals and reducing pain (such as *hong hua* 红花, *dang gui* 当归, *chuan xiong* 川芎, *chi shao* 赤芍 and *tao ren* 桃仁) repeatedly showed up as the most frequently used herbs of clinical trials for post-stroke shoulder disorders.

Summary of Chinese Herbal Medicine Clinical Evidence

Among the three commonly seen shoulder complications, SHS has been the most investigated by clinical trials of CHM. This is in contrast to the relatively small number of studies identified in shoulder pain and shoulder subluxation. For example, only three studies utilising some forms of topical CHM targeting shoulder subluxation were included in our evaluation. With regard to managing the shoulder pain, CHM, especially topical CHM, has been studied and proved beneficial when used as an add-on therapy. Once SHS develops, the treatment usually involves a more complex symptom control method and requires longer duration. CHMs of both oral and topical administration are likely to help at this stage, in particular when used as an add-on therapy to routine rehabilitation.

Evaluation of the clinical study evidence found variation in formulas and routes of administration of CHM, and diversity in outcomes reported. Topical CHM was the most frequently investigated CHM, being used in the majority of studies. The treatment duration varied from ten days to three months. Chinese medicine syndrome differentiation is not the highlight of clinical studies, since the majority of studies all selected similar treatment principles and herbs. Although no known CHM formula has been repeatedly evaluated according to the formula name, based on the herb ingredients, it could be summarized that the Blood-moving herbs are the most frequently used ones.

In terms of the treatment effects, some promising clinical evidence was seen with oral CHM, topical CHM and the combination of oral and topical CHM for all the three types of post-stroke shoulder complications. It is noted that topical CHM may play the most important role in the management of post-stroke shoulder complications.

For post-stroke shoulder subluxation, topically used CHM steam therapy and fomentation may reduce the pain of shoulder joints, and improve the shoulder function and the patients' daily activities. However, it is not clear whether CHM could reduce the subluxation itself, since the studies did not report on this particular outcome. As for post-stroke shoulder pain, a single study suggested that oral CHM targeting pain symptoms (*Shen tong zhu yu tang* 身痛逐瘀汤) is effective for pain score and also patients' daily activities when it was integrated with routine rehabilitation therapy. Topical CHM used as fomentation and steam therapy both are beneficial for reducing pain score and improving the shoulder function. For the management of SHS, meta-analysis showed that *Bu yang huan wu tang* 补阳还五汤 could effectively reduce pain symptoms. All four topical CHM forms (CHM bath therapy, fomentation, CHM steam therapy and CHM external application) have been evaluated when used as integrative medicine. All these are beneficial for pain symptoms and shoulder function, while fomentation and CHM bath therapy were evidenced as being effective to improve patients' daily activities. However, there is no particular formula which is confirmed as the most effective, although all unnamed formulas have some herbs in common.

Herbs used both orally and topically that may have contributed to the positive effects include *chuan xiong* 川芎, *hong hua* 红花, *dang gui* 当归, *chi shao* 赤芍, *gui zhi* 桂枝 and *sang zhi* 桑枝. Some herbs are more often used topically; using them this way has contributed to the positive effects. These are *shen jin cao* 伸筋草, *tou gu cao* 透骨草, *mo yao* 没药 and *ru xiang* 乳香. Practitioners may consider these herbs when preparing prescriptions for patients with post-stroke shoulder complications. Few side effects were reported, with CHM considered to be safe for post-stroke shoulder complications based on included studies.

Assessment using GRADE methods found that although significant benefit of adding topical CHM to routine rehabilitation was found in all three complications, the evidence certainty was assessed as 'low' or 'very low'. The main reasons for quality downgrading are lack of blinding, heterogeneity of analyses and small sample size.

As no minimal clinically important difference has been determined for the outcomes in post-stroke shoulder complications, the clinical relevance of findings remains uncertain. In terms of the outcome measures used by clinical studies, effective rate was the most commonly reported one. Due to the lack of consistent criteria for effective rate calculation, it is difficult to interpret these results. In fact, the shoulder complications are closely related to pain, patients' upper limb function and therefore affecting patients' daily activity. Further studies should consider using a group of outcome measures to reflect treatment effects in different perspectives. In addition, for shoulder subluxation, the outcome measure of Acromiohumeral interval (AHI), which specifically measures the shoulder joint pathologies, could be selected.

It will be interesting to know when CHM treatment should start after the onset of stroke. However, such information was not particularly reported by included clinical studies.

Mild adverse events caused by oral CHM were rarely reported and adverse events caused by topical CHM were not seen. Topical CHM has been shown as an effective and safe therapy for post-stroke shoulder complications; it seems more commonly used than oral CHM in clinical studies.

In summary, there is promising evidence supporting the use of CHM for the management of post-stroke shoulder complications, in particular the topical use of CHM. Clinical practice may consider incorporating therapies of bath, steam, fomentation and topical application of CHM in routine rehabilitation as the management of post-stroke shoulder complications.

References

1. Perrin M, Ramelet AA. (2011) Pharmacological treatment of primary chronic venous disease: Rationale, results and unanswered questions. *Eur J Vasc Endovasc Surg* **41**(1): 117–125.

References to Included Studies

Study No.	References
H1	黄开学, 杨芳, 张宗美, 徐立新, 徐贞杰, 郭强, 王义亮. (2012) 运动疗法联合中药薰蒸治疗脑卒中肩关节半脱位. 中国康复 (1): 42683.
H2	覃素娟, 黎敏平. (2014) 中药烫疗联合早期康复治疗脑卒中肩关节半脱位 37 例. 甘肃中医学院学报 (3): 53–55.

(Continued)

(Continued)

Study No.	References
H3	郭友华, 朱乐英, 詹乐昌, 陈红霞. (2013) 四子散热敷配合康复训练治疗中风后肩痛 30 例疗效观察. 新中医 (9): 130–131.
H4	杨雅琴. (2008) 综合康复治疗脑卒中后肩关节半脱位的疗效观察. 华中医学杂志 (2): 109–110.
H5	陈德仁. (2011) 身痛逐瘀汤加减配合康复训练治疗脑卒中后肩痛 35 例临床观察. 中国疗养医学 (10): 883–884.
H6	洪敏巧, 李灵萍, 李秀彬,. (2012) 中药包热敷配合康复训练治疗脑卒中后肩痛的疗效观察. 浙江中医杂志 (5): 328.
H7	刘新, 戚小航, 吴昊, 蒋苹, 杨轶楠. (2015) 综合康复训练治疗偏瘫后肩痛的临床观察. 中国中医急症 (4): 720–722.
H8	陈健云, 张国庆, 周湘明, 曹德付. (2012) 中药熏蒸结合Bobath疗法治疗脑卒中偏瘫后肩痛疗效观察. 苏州大学学报·医学版 (2): 267–268.
H9	郭静华, 王艳华. (2012)骨刺消痛液热敷联合中频电及运动疗法治疗脑卒中后肩痛疗效观察. 现代中西医结合杂志 (27): 2998–2999.
H10	吴春苗. (2012) 中药湿热敷配合综合康复治疗中风后偏瘫肩痛的病例观察. 中国现代医生 (19): 80–82.
H11	佟飞. (2013) 中药溻渍治疗卒中偏瘫后肩痛 32 例疗效观察. 河北中医 (3): 351–352.
H12	王康锋, 杨军. (2013) 中药透皮给药结合康复促通技术治疗卒中后肩痛疗效观察. 中国中医药信息杂志 (9): 68–69.
H13	杨军, 王康锋. (2013) 中药透皮给药结合康复促通技术治疗卒中后肩痛疗效观察. 山东中医药杂志 (9): 626–627.
H14	彭银英, 朱乐英. (2013) 中药局部熏蒸治疗偏瘫肩痛的临床疗效观察. 广州中医药大学学报 (1): 16–18.
H15	张忠霞, 张学玲, 高汉义. (2011) 中药熏洗加运动疗法治疗脑卒中偏瘫后肩痛疗效观察. 山东医药 (33): 98–99.
H16	赵英, 王晓敏. (2005) 中药熏蒸加Bobath运动疗法治疗偏瘫性肩痛疗效观察. 内蒙古中医药 (6): 23–24.
H17	陈宗华, 黄宗菊, 肖慈丽, 杨小梅. (2013) 中药熏蒸配合运动疗法治疗偏瘫后肩痛临床研究. 实用中医药杂志 (2): 80–81.
H18	杨丽. (2015) 中药熨烫配合康复训练治疗脑卒中肩关节疼痛效果观察. 湖北中医杂志 (2): 47–48.

(Continued)

Study No.	References
H19	高小溪. (2011) 综合康复治疗脑卒中后肩痛 40 例疗效观察. 中国冶金工业医学杂志 (1): 60–61.
H20	左永发, 韩淑凯, 张宝昌. (2010) 补气化痰通络法结合康复疗法治疗脑卒中后 I 期肩手综合征临床观察. 中国中医急症 (4): 555571.
H21	孟长君,李春华, 王德生, 张永刚. (2009) 补阳还五汤合五苓散配合康复治疗卒中后肩手综合征临床观察. 中国中医急症 (6): 872–873.
H22	柳淑青. (2011) 补阳还五汤加味治疗卒中后肩手综合征疗效观察. 四川中医 (11): 81–82.
H23	唐武, 李庆. (2013) 傅青主两臂肩膊痛方加减治疗卒中后肩手综合征 36 例临床观察. 中医药导报 (3): 49–50.
H24	贾爱明, 胡文梅, 张红, 刘耘, 董玉宽, 刁凤声, 毕伟莲, 艾群. (2013) 加味补阳还五汤联合康复训练对脑卒中后急性期肩手综合征的疗效. 广东医学 (12): 1933–1935.
H25	薛艺东. (2008) 加味补阳还五汤配合神经功能康复训练治疗卒中后肩手综合征. 中西医结合心脑血管病杂志 (5): 621–622.
H26	段红莉, 王雅娟, 刘玉洁. (2009) 芍药甘草汤加减治疗卒中后肩手综合征 36 例. 陕西中医 (9): 1160–1161.
H27	李文杰, 张方. (2009) 通络活血汤加康复训练治疗中风后肩手综合征 60 例. 实用中西医结合临床 (2): 15–16.
H28	许幸仪, 黄坚红, 黄德弘, 刘健红, 王成银, 王春雷. (2013) 益肾解痉汤联合常规康复疗法治疗脑卒中后肩手综合征 30 例临床观察. 中医杂志 (23): 2012–2014 & 2045.
H29	杨伟红, 杨光福, ,韩淑凯. (2011) 针药结合治疗脑卒中后肩手综合征疗效观察. 中国中医急症 (9): 1404–1405 & 1412.
H30	张燕龙, 张方. (2011) 中西医结合及康复训练治疗中风后肩手综合征 60 例. 中国中医急症 (9): 1473–1474.
H31	陆树列. (2013) 中西医结合及康复训练综合治疗中风后肩手综合征疗效观察. 亚太传统医药 (4): 80–81.
H32	占戈, 田园. (2007) 中西医结合治疗脑卒中后肩手综合征 I 期的临床观察. 北京中医 (9): 589–591.
H33	高震. (2008) 中药配合康复疗法治疗脑卒中后肩手综合征疗效观察. 实用中医药杂志 (1): 6.

(Continued)

(*Continued*)

Study No.	References
H34	陈德仁. (2012) 中药配合康复训练治疗脑卒中后肩手综合征 30 例临床观察. 中国疗养医学 (3): 205–206.
H35	王雷, 孙波. (2011) 自拟培土舒痛汤对 I 期肩手综合征临床疗效观察. 光明中医 (12): 2437–2438.
H36	陈建勇, 李华, 黎京京. (2014) 综合治疗中风偏瘫后肩手综合征 35 例临床观察. 湖南中医杂志 (3): 40–41.
H37	王著敏, 金杰, 王荣珠. (2006) 分期辨治脑卒中后肩手综合征 100 例. 现代中医药 (5): 15–16.
H38	杨进. 马勇. (2012) 益肾蠲痹汤治疗脑卒中后肩手综合征 26 例. 河南中医 (5): 610–611.
H39	郭知学, 李欧, 周末法, 王圣祥. (2008) 中西医结合治疗脑卒中后肩手综合征. 现代中西医结合杂志 (24): 3813–3814.
H40	陈晓枫, 赖清只, 程熙, 卢金华, 高燕玲. (2014) 加味金黄散配合康复训练治疗中风后肩手综合征的临床随机对照试验. 内蒙古中医药 (32): 42684.
H41	张航, 陈默, 支英豪, 叶茜茜, 项玉央. (2010) 金黄膏外敷配合康复训练治疗脑卒中肩手综合征 30 例. 中国中医急症 (4): 676–677.
H42	陈艳军, 安文灿, 金莉. (2015) 康复功能训练配合中药泡洗治疗中风病肩手综合征 50 例观察. 实用中医药杂志 (3): 193–194.
H43	郭友华, 陈红霞, 杨志敬, 李梅. (2011) 冷热中药交替浸浴疗法结合康复训练治疗脑卒中后肩手综合征的疗效观察. 中华物理医学与康复杂志 (4): 303–304.
H44	刘惠惠. (2013) 冷热中药交替浸浴疗法结合康复训练治疗脑卒中后肩手综合征的效果分析. 中外医疗 (24): 139–140.
H45	耿润华, 范传廷. (2005) 脑卒中后肩手综合征早期疼痛中西医康复的临床研究. 中华实用中西医杂志 **18**(3): 334–335.
H46	余恒旺, 崔美莲, 梁思杰, 聂志华, 颜冬润, 李凯凤. (2006) 舒筋活络散治疗脑卒中后肩手综合征临床观察. 中国中医急症 (9): 942–943.
H47	朱乐英, 彭银英. (2009) 舒筋活络洗剂浸浴治疗中风后肩手综合征 26 例疗效观察. 新中医 (2): 57–58.
H48	吴海科, 顾卫, 谭峰, 王金良, 黄涛, 张明霞. (2004) 舒筋洗药治疗脑卒中后肩手综合征 42 例. 中医外治杂志 (6): 11.

(*Continued*)

Study No.	References
H49	包艳, 刘海兰, 周晓燕, 陈晓峰, 蔡超群. (2013) 五苓散冷热浸泡结合康复训练对脑卒中后肩手综合征患者的影响. 护士进修杂志 (24): 2269–2270.
H50	邹丽萍, 林娟. (2011) 五子散结合电脑中频治疗肩手综合征效果观察. 中国中医药咨讯 (23): 135.
H51	李玉岭, 闫国庆. (2007) 药浴结合运动疗法治疗脑卒中后肩手综合征疗效分析. 中西医结合心脑血管病杂志 (1): 75.
H52	阙建兰, 边雪梅, 裘涛, 陈眉. (2012) 中药局部加压熏蒸治疗肩手综合征 40 例临床观察. 中医杂志 (12): 1035–1037.
H53	朱坚, 许建平. (2015) 中药泡洗联合康复训练治疗中风恢复期肩手综合征临床观察. 中国中医急症 (2): 363–365.
H54	朱宏勋, 邹忆怀. (2008) 中药泡洗治疗脑卒中后肩手综合征的临床疗效观察. 中国康复医学杂志 (9): 845–846.
H55	赵超蓉, 郑超英, 周芸, 黄旭. (2014) 中药泡洗治疗中风病恢复期肩手综合征疗效观察. 中国中医急症 (1): 39–41.
H56	安国英, 闫文革. (2012) 中药热敷联合空气波压力治疗仪治疗脑卒中后肩手综合征的疗效观察. 中华中医药杂志 (8): 2118–2119.
H57	郭健. 刘娇. (2011) 中药热奄包配合康复训练治疗卒中后肩手综合征的疗效观察. 中医临床研究 (20): 13–14.
H58	吕畅. (2013) 中药湿热敷配合康复训练治疗肩手综合征的疗效观察. 内蒙古中医药 (35): 39.
H59	韦华军. (2010) 中药穴位热敷疗法治疗脑卒中后肩手综合征. 中国社区医师·医学专业 (3): 85–86.
H60	王艳昕, 蔡永亮, 许珍晶, 徐磊. (2011) 中药熏洗和肩封治疗中风后肩手综合征 48 例. 中医药临床杂志 (12): 1075–1077.
H61	杨军, 孙灵芝. (2011) 中药熏洗结合促通技术治疗脑卒中后肩手综合征 60 例. 中国医药导报 (3): 83–84.
H62	高广林. (2013) 中药熏洗结合康复训练治疗肩手综合征 60 例临床观察. 中国社区医师·医学专业 (10): 225–226.
H63	徐素美, 张超. (2011) 中药熏蒸辅治脑梗死后肩手综合征. 浙江中西医结合杂志 (7): 500–501.
H64	马振宇, 吴赞杨. (2013) 中药熏蒸结合pnf技术治疗脑卒中后肩手综合征 I 期疗效观察. 浙江中西医结合杂志 (8): 623–625.

(Continued)

(Continued)

Study No.	References
H65	林任. 陈丽丽. (2014) 中药熏蒸联合肢体康复训练对脑梗死后肩手综合征患者疼痛、水肿及肩手功能活动的影响. 河南中医 (7): 1282–1283.
H66	秦剑剑, 秦德宝, 闫玮娟, 孙珊珊. (2014) 中药熏蒸疗法治疗脑卒中肩手综合征的临床疗效观察. 中国疗养医学 (9): 806–807.
H67	涂颖廷, 李丰兰, 王长青. (2010) 中药熏蒸治疗中风后肩手综合征 23 例. 中医外治杂志 (5): 22–23.
H68	贺青涛. (2011) 中药药熨结合康复训练治疗脑卒中后肩手综合征的临床观察. 按摩与康复医学 (5): 200–201.
H69	罗彩花, 贺青涛, 聂斌, 王慧, 王俊华. (2008) 中药熨结合康复训练干预脑卒中后肩手综合征的临床研究. 中西医结合心脑血管病杂志 (8): 907–909.
H70	龙美丽. (2013) 中药熨烫联合早期功能锻炼对中风后肩手综合征的效果. 护理实践与研究 (12): 25–26.
H71	谭璐璐, 陈兴华. (2015) '通络Ⅰ方' 辨证取穴烫熨治疗脑梗死后肩手综合征Ⅰ期临床疗效. 辽宁中医杂志 (3): 526–528.
H72	林琴. (2014) 红花酒精涂擦结合十一方药渣熨治疗中风后肩手综合征 30 例. 中医外治杂志 (4): 20–21.
H73	王瑞平. (2012) 三联疗法治疗脑卒中后肩手综合征的临床疗效观察. 中国实用神经疾病杂志 (18): 54–55.
H74	朱宏勋. (2003) 中药泡洗结合功能训练对脑卒中后肩手综合征的临床研究 [D]. 北京中医药大学.
H75	詹乐昌, 陈红霞, 谢仁明, 欧海宁. (2010) 中西医结合康复治疗中风后肩手综合征 40 例疗效观察. 中华中医药学刊 (12): 2526–2527.
H76	潘德祥, 张雯, 金海涛. (2010) 中药熏洗治疗脑卒中后肩手综合征 80 例. 中医外治杂志 (1): 32–33.
H77	芦玉莲, 陈文卫. (2007) 中药薰蒸配合运动疗法治疗脑卒中后肩手综合征 36 例分析. 中国现代医药杂志 (12): 105–106.
H78	刘玉香, 黄宝琴, 何丽卿. (2005) 脑卒中后肩手综合征中医药综合康复护理体会. 中华临床医学研究杂志 (12): 1752–1753.
H79	张颖, 沈俊, 王毓雯. (2006) 中药熏蒸结合运动疗法治疗早期肩手综合症临床观察. 中华临床医学研究杂志 (20): 2706.
H80	袁威, 赵振. (2010) 综合疗法治疗脑卒中后肩手综合征 38 例疗效观察. 国医论坛 (6): 27–28.

(Continued)

(Continued)

Study No.	References
H81	王春霞. (2013) 温阳通络法治疗中风后肩手综合征 90 例临床研究. 中国实用医药 (6): 169–170.
H82	王红燕. (2011) 星状神经节阻滞联合中药治疗肩手综合征 40 例. 心血管病防治知识 (学术版) (1): 34–35.
H83	赵欣. (2013) 中药内外并治脑卒中后肩手综合征的临床疗效观察 [D]. 湖南中医药大学.

6

Pharmacological Actions of the Common Herbs

OVERVIEW

The therapeutic effects of Chinese herbal medicine for post-stroke shoulder complications are due to the activity of the chemical compounds they contain. This section reviews the available experimental evidence to explain the possible biological activity of the ten most frequently used Chinese herbs from randomised clinical trials presented in Chapter 5.

Introduction

Chinese herbal formulas and herbs exert their actions through active constituent compounds. Clinical trials assess the efficacy and safety of formulas and herbs; however, trials do not usually investigate herbal mechanisms of action. Experimental studies including *in vitro* and *in vivo* research investigate potential mechanisms of herbs.

This chapter includes experimental cell and animal model evidence for the top ten herbs identified in Chapter 5. The most frequently used herbs are *hong hua* 红花, *gui zhi* 桂枝, *dang gui* 当归, *chuan xiong* 川芎, *tou gu cao* 透骨草, *mu gua* 木瓜, *huang qi* 黄芪, *bai shao* 白芍, *sang zhi* 桑枝, and *tao ren* 桃仁. Of these herbs, *tou gu cao* and *shen jin cao* were most frequently used topically, whilst the remaining herbs were used both topically or orally. This chapter provides biological plausibility and possible explanations for the positive findings shown in clinical trials.

Experimental Studies on *hong hua*

Hong hua 红花 (*Carthamus tinctorius* L.) consists predominantly of quinochalcones, flavonoids, alkaloids, polyacetylene, aromatic glucosides and organic acids.[1] The quinochalcones and flavonoids are considered to be *hong hua*'s most characteristic and active constituents, with quinochalcone hydroxysafflor yellow A (HSYA) and flavonoid kaempferol reported as the primarily bioactive component.[2,3]

Methanol extracts of *hong hua* have shown to be anti-inflammatory, inducing heme oxygenase-1 in lipopolysaccharide (LPS) activated macrophages. Induction subsequently inhibits inducible nitric oxide synthase (iNOS) and cyclooxygenase (COX)-2, leading to reductions in production of nitric oxide (NO) and prostaglandin E2 (PGE2). Methanol extract of *hong hua* also reduces nuclear factor kappa-light-chain-enhancer of activated B cells (NF-κB) binding and luciferase activity, and inhibits tumor necrosis factor (TNF)-alpha mediated vascular cell adhesion molecule (VCAM)-1 expression.[4] These activities may reduce peripheral damage in the local shoulder area.

Water extract of *hong hua* has shown to be neuroprotective to stroke-affected areas. In a C6 glia cell death model, water extract enhances scavenging of hydroxyl and 1,1-diphenyl-2-picrylhydrazyl (DPPH) radicals, inhibiting cell death. Furthermore, in mouse cerebrum, water extract decreases malondialdehyde formation. In mouse cerebral cortex injected with ferrous chloride (FeCl(3)) solution, water extract prevents increases in thiobarbituric acid reactive substances and 8-hydroxy-2′-deoxyguanosine (8-OHdG).[5]

In haemorheological mouse and rat models, *hong hua* water extract inhibits thrombosis development, and when combined with clopidogrel, reduces overall venous thrombus weight and prolongs prothombin time. In a pulmonary embolism, model extract also reduces the paralysis of animals injected with collagen and epinephrine.[6]

In isoprenaline-induced ischaemic rat models, a manufactured *hong hua* extract showed anti-inflammatory effects by reducing interleukin (IL)-6 and TNF-α in serum and suppressing Bax protein expression.[7]

An extract of *hong hua*, known as carthamus yellow, is a common food colour and flavour additive with experimental evidence relevant to stroke disease.[8] In rats placed in ice water and injected with epinephrine, carthamus yellow inhibits blood viscosity and erythrocyte aggregation. Such activity is dose dependent, showing a delay in prothombin time and reduced aggregation of haematocrit and platelets.[9] In LPS-activated macrophages, carthamus yellow inhibits NO, PGE2 and IL-1b release, likely by attenuating iNOS and COX-2 expression, without suppressing NF-κB phosphorylation.[10]

Hydroxysafflor yellow A has also shown to be cytoprotective and to show antiplatelet activity. In a hypoxic endothelial cell model, HYSA enhances the survival of cells by inhibiting apoptosis, upregulating bcl-2/bax ratio and increasing vascular endothelial growth factor (VEGF) protein concentration.[11] Such activity may benefit stroke-affected tissue by reducing infarct area and inhibiting neuron damage from glutamate exposure.[12] A study in brain injured rats supports the neuroprotective potential of HYSA, showing that it attenuates neural cell apoptosis and alleviates neurological symptoms by inhibiting endothelial nitric oxide synthase (eNOS) and decreasing mRNA and its protein expression.[13]

In rabbit platelets and polymorphonuclear leukocytes, HYSA inhibits their aggregation, indicating its antiplatelet activity.[14]

Individual constituents of *hong hua* have also shown some limited antioxidative and anti-inflammatory activity. In an ischaemic guinea pig heart model, N-(p-Coumaroyl)serotonin raises NO levels, increasing antioxidant activity and protecting myocardial function.[15] In carrageenan-induced rats, the saponin, 3β-O-[β-D-xylopyranosyl (1 → 3)-O-β-D-galactopyranosyl]-lup-12-ene-28 oic acid-28-O-α-L-rhamnopyranosyl este, reduces oedema paw volume; however, the mechanisms are unclear.[16]

Experimental Studies on *gui zhi*

*Gui zhi*桂枝 has a number of common sources including *Cinnamomum cassia* Presl, *Cinnamomum tamala* and *Cinnamomum burmannii*.[17]

Component compounds are predominantly aromatics, diterpenes and polyphenols, with cinnamic acid, cinnamaldehyde, enzoic acid, cinnamyl alcohol and coumarin common biomarkers.[17,18]

Dimethyl sulfoxide extract of *gui zhi* has been investigated for muscle dystrophy in human skin fibroblast NB1RGB cells.[19] Collagen contains high amounts of substrates important for creatine synthesis and muscle regeneration, improving muscle strength.[20,21] By increasing phosphorylation of insulin-like growth factor (IGF)-1 receptor and downstream signalling molecules, including insulin receptor substrate-1 and extracellular signal-regulated kinases (Erk)1/2, *gui zhi* extract enhances collagen production.[19]

A study in LPS-stimulated murine peritoneal macrophages shows cinnamaldehyde is a potent inhibitor of NO production.[22] In a middle cerebral artery occlusion mouse model, cinnamaldehyde reduces neurological deficit scores, neural oedema and infarct volume. Mechanistically, cinnamaldehyde suppresses activation of toll-like receptor 4, TNF-α receptor associated factor 6 and NF-κB. This subsequently suppresses a rise in TNF-α, IL-1β, CCL2 and endothelial-leukocyte adhesion molecule-1, thus reducing ischaemic leukocyte infiltration.[23] A similar study in LPS-induced BV-2 microglial cells decreased iNOS and COX-2 protein expression levels and suppressed nuclear translocation of NF-κB p65 and p50.[24] Topically though, the effects of cinnamaldehyde have shown to be anti-therapeutic in mouse ears. Cinnamaldehyde application induces inflammation and cellular infiltration, likely by stimulating transient receptor potential cation channel (TRPA1).[25] Such inflammation can stimulate itch response when topically applied to human skin.[26]

Experimental Studies on *dang gui*

The main *dang gui* 当归 source is *Angelica sinensis* and its constituent content predominantly consists of ferulic acid, Z-ligustilide, butylidenephthalide, senkyunolide I, senkyunolide H and coniferyl ferulate.[27,28]

In a rodent carotid artery occlusion model, *Angelica sinensis* extract enhances hippocampal neurogenesis and restores brain-derived neurotrophic factor (BDNF) expression. In addition, the extract reverses the decreases in phosphorylation of cyclic adenosine monophosphate (cAMP)-responsive element binding protein (CREB).[29]

In a rat artery occlusion model, ferulic acid suppresses superoxide radicals and reduces intercellular adhesion molecule (ICAM)-1 and NF-κB expression, reducing the size of cerebral infarct and neurological deficit.[30] A similar ischaemic study shows a general downregulation in inflammation by ferulic acid, by reducing caspase-3 expression, decreasing ICAM-1 mRNA levels and decreasing microglia/macrophages.[31] A more recent ischaemic occlusion model indicates ferulic acid also attenuates hippocampal nerve injury and increases the erythropoietin content of peripheral blood.[32] Investigating ferulic acid in rat viability of Schwann cells, shows that it significantly increases the number of proliferating Schwann cells and enhances their regeneration rate, whilst decreasing macrophage recruitment. Significantly shorter latency and accelerated nerve conductive velocity are physiological effects of such activity, which shows potential therapeutic benefit for peripheral nerve injury.[33] These activities likely contribute to the neurogenic action of *dang gui* extract.

Beyond ferulic acid's neurogenic and inflammatory potential, there is also limited evidence of it cardiovascular protective benefits. In hypertensive rats, ferulic acid decreases plasma angiotensin-1-converting enzyme (ACE) activity with a reduction in blood pressure. Biologically, mRNA expression of genes associated with lipid metabolism are downregulated and total cholesterol and triglyceride levels are reduced.[34] This has potential for stroke prevention interventions.

Ligustilide, a major constituent of *dang gui*, is known to permeate the blood-brain barrier (BBB).[35] In a forebrain ischaemic rat model, it enhances cognitive function and protects the hippocampus.[36] In an ischaemic occlusion rat model, a ligustilide dose dependently reduces brain swelling and improves deficits in behaviour.[37] A subarachnoid haemorrhage rat model also shows that ligustilide reduces the incidence of cerebral vasospasm and mortality.[38] These physiological benefits could be due to a reduction in apoptotic cells in the injured area via the downregulation of proapoptotic proteins, p53, and cleaved caspase-3. Further explanation of effects could be that ligustilide induces Nrf2 nuclear translocation, upregulates heme oxygenase (HO)-1 expression and strengthens BBB permeability.[38] In a rat artery occlusion model, ligustilide has been shown in the parietal cortex and hippocampus to prevent neuronal loss, dendrite damage and neuronal apoptosis whilst also inhibiting astrocyte activation and proliferation.[39]

Following a stroke, adipose-derived stem cells have therapeutic potential for rescuing damaged tissue. Ligustilide treatment, in a study of mice transplanted with adipose-derived stem cells, improved the efficacy of transplantation.[40]

A number of vascular-related activities have been associated with *dang gui* constituent, butylidenephthalide. In cultured mouse aorta smooth muscle cells, derivatives of butylidenephthalide have shown to be anti-proliferative.[41] In animal and human platelet models, butylidenephthalide inhibits platelet aggregation, possibly by inhibiting cyclo-oxygenase.[42] In inflamed rat brain, stimulated by LPS, butylidenephthalide reduces hippocampal cell neurodegeneration by regulating chronic microglial activation and inhibiting production of NO, TNF-α and IL-1b.[43] A hybrid DL-3-n-butylphthalide has approval from the State Food and Drug Administration (SFDA) of China for clinical use in stroke patients. Research of the synthesised compound shows reductions in oxidative stress and neuronal apoptosis, and improves memory and learning deficits.[44]

Senkyunolide I passes the BBB in rats and opens tight junctions to allow other compounds to permeate.[45,46] In a rat cerebral occlusion model, senkyunolide I improves neurological deficit, reduces infarct volume and limits cerebral oedema. Furthermore, malondialdehyde (MDA) levels decreased, superoxide dismutase activity increased, Bcl-2/Bax ratio improved and the expression of cleaved caspase 3 and 9 was inhibited.[47]

Experimental Studies on *chuan xiong*

Commonly sourced from *Ligusticum chuanxiong* Hort., *chuan xiong's* 川芎 main constituents include ferulic acid, senkyunolide I, senkyunolide H, senkyunolide A, ligustilide, levistolide A and cafeic acid (phenolic).[48,49]

Ferulic acid, senkyunolide I and ligustilide act in the same way as *dang gui* with regard to stroke-related activity (see *dang gui* section). In LPS-induced murine microglial cells, a fraction of *Ligusticum chuanxiong* has been shown to be a potent inhibitor of nitrate production. High-performance liquid chromatography (HPLC) identifies that senkyunolide A and Z-ligustilide make up the majority of this active fraction. These compounds inhibit induction of TNF-α and, via inhibition of inflammatory mediators, protect Neuro-2a cell cultures from cytotoxicity. Action on TNF-α is likely through reducing the stability of TNF-a mRNA.[50] In an *in vitro* model, senkyunolide I, senkyunolide A and ligustilide have been shown to enhance the transport of another botanical compound (paeoniflorin) through the BBB.[46]

Extracted from *chuan xiong*, tetramethylpyrazine (TMP) has research indicating it can assist in stroke damage minimalisation. In a rat cerebral occlusion model, TMP has shown to be anti-inflammatory and neuroprotective, reducing infarct size, decreasing cerebral oedema and preserving neurons.[51] In SH-SY5Y cells, TMP stimulates neuronal differentiation.[52] The proliferation and differentiation of neural stem cells into neurons in hypoxic rat brain by TMP may be due to increased phosphorylation of ERK and changes to p38.[53] A study in wound healing shows TMP not only promotes neural precursor cell migration, but also enhances such migration to ischaemic regions.[54]

In brain endothelial cells, there is increased autocrine signalling of VEGF following TMP administration.[55] In rats, TMP also reduces platelet aggregation and blood viscosity.[56]

Due to its neuroprotective activity in microglial cells, chrysophanol is another compound which may be of interest for stroke, although its research is limited and the bioavailability in *chuan xiong* is unclear.[57]

Experimental Studies on *tou gu cao*

Tou gu cao 透骨草 is primarily sourced from *Speranskia tuberculata* (*Bunge*) Baill. or *Impatiens balsamina* L., but there is regional variation.[58]

Compounds 18-hydroxy(-)-manool and beta-sitosterol have been extracted from *Speranskia tuberculata,* as well as a number of alkaloids, speranskatines A and B, and speranculatines A-C.[59–60] However, there has not been any published research exploring their biological activity related to stroke.

Impatiens balsamina consists predominantly of benzopyrones, benzofuranones, naphthoquinones, alkaloids and flavonoids with kaempferol, quercetin and lawsone having the greatest bio-availability.[61,62]

A published review on biological activity of kaempferol indicates it is a potent anti-inflammatory agent.[63] Kaempferol and quercetin have similar structures and mechanisms; in cultured human umbilical vein endothelial cells, both inhibit inflammatory mediator COX-2, the blockade of NF-κB and activator protein-1.[64] Furthermore, both reduce expression of endothelial adhesion molecules such as (ICAM)-1 and VCAM-1.[64]

Another compound, of lesser bioavailability, but also exhibiting COX-2 inhibition, is 1,4-naphthoquinones.[65]

Experimental Studies on *mu gua*

A number of species of *Chaenomeles* are sourced for *mu gua* 木瓜, with their fruit portion the medicinal component consisting predominantly of flavonols, oligomers and triterpenes.

Flavonols, epicatechin and procyanidin have the greatest bio-availability, with oleanolic acid and ursolic acid the greatest of the tritepenes.[66,67] Extracts of *Chaenomeles cathayensis* and *Chaenomeles thibetica* have shown to be strong antioxidants with research indicating proanthocyanidin constituents are likely responsible.[67,68] Proanthocyanidins have been proposed to reduce cardiovascular disease risk, which may have benefits for stroke prevention.[69] *In vitro/in vivo* rat experiments show *Chaenomeles thibetica* extracts prevent oxidative liver damage, with less circulating aspartate aminotransferase (AST) and alanine aminotransferase (ALT) evidenced.[70] Extract also inhibits COX-1 and COX-2 enzymes, with extract components incorporated into lipid membranes thus hindering the diffusion of free radicals and reducing oxidative reactions and lipid peroxidation.[71] In mouse LPS models, ethnolic extracts have also shown antioxidant activity by inhibiting NO production, as well as gene induction of TNF-α, interferon gamma (IFN-γ) and granulocyte-colony stimulating factor (G-CSF).[72]

Contained glucoside fractions of *Chaenomeles* in a rat model of arthritis reduce paw swelling and pain response.[73] In peritoneal macrophages, the fraction reduces lymphocyte proliferation, IL-2 production and levels of IL-1 and TNF-α.[74] In S180 tumour-transplanted mice, a water-soluble polysaccharide from *Chaenomeles* is immune stimulating, which may have benefits for macrophage phagocytosis and may speed up tissue recovery in stroke patients.[75]

The anti-inflammatory activity of extracts may be due to 3,4-dihydroxybenzoic acid content, inhibiting DPPH and possibly production of TNF-α.[76]

In cultured cortical rat neurons, oleanolic acid has shown neuronal cell-specific antioxidant activity, inhibiting cell death from hydrogen peroxide and reducing reactive oxygen species (ROS) generation.[77] Oleanolic acid effects have shown to prolong mice survival time in an cerebral artery occlusion ischaemia model.[78] In an ischaemic model, oleanolic acid promotes activation of nuclear factor-erythroid 2-related factor 2, and decreases toll-like receptor4 and NF-αB expression.[79]

Ursolic acid may be of use for cardiovascular conditions, as in rabbit atria administered isoproterenol, it decreases peptide secretion and cAMP levels.[80] This may have benefit for improving cardiovascular homeostasis and reducing stroke risk.

Experimental Studies on *huang qi*

The official source of *huang qi* 黄芪 is *Astragalus membranaceus*, and the primary bioactive component of its roots are astragalosides, calycosin and calycosin-7-O-β-d-glucoside.[81]

A human study of *Astragalus membranaceus* extract for acute haemorrhagic stroke, compared to placebo, shows it improves the Glasgow outcome scale score.[82] Clinical improvement in stroke has been proposed to be due to the neuroprotective activity of contained compounds. In a rat focal cerebral ischaemic model, extract combined with ligustrazine reinforces the BBB and alleviates microhaemorrhage.[83] In HepG2 cells stimulated with TNF-α, extracts have shown anti-inflammatory activity, dose-dependently inhibiting NF-κB activation and the expression of iNOS and ICAM-1 mRNA.[84]

Astragaloside IV has therapeutic potential for stroke, with a review of the literature indicating diverse potential neuroprotective and cardioprotective pathway activity.[85] In an ischaemic cerebral rat model, possibly via the regulation of junctional proteins, astragaloside IV attenuates BBB permeability.[86] Furthermore, an ischemia/reperfusion rat study shows upregulation of matrix metalloproteinase (MMP)-9 and aquaporin (AQP)4 is inhibited by astragaloside IV, with a subsequent reduction of oedema and tissue damage.[84] In a subarachnoid haemorrhagic rat model, astragaloside IV increases malondialdehyde, decreases neuronal apoptosis and reduces the presence of cleaved caspase-3 and superoxide dismutase activity in ischaemic tissue.[87] However, there is evidence from rat and dog studies that suggest astragaloside IV may have difficulty passing the BBB.[88]

There have been reports of calycosin having potential neuroprotective and anti-inflammatory benefits for stroke.[89] In a rat cerebral artery occlusion model, calycosin reduces neurological deficit and infarct volume, reduces malondialdehyde and ROS, and upregulates superoxide dismutase activity.[90] An occlusion model shows it may also downregulate RASD1 and upregulate oestrogen receptor-α, miR-375 and Bcl-2.[91] From a cerebral artery occlusion model in rats, calycosin's neuroprotective activity is likely via inhibition of MMP (MMP-2 and MMP-9) expression and activity, scavenging of NO and subsequently reducing cell death.[92] Interestingly, in a myocardial ischaemic rat model, by enhancing VEGF mRNA and protein expression, calycosin promotes angiogenesis.[93]

Experimental Studies on *bai shao*

The main botanical source for *bai shao* 白芍 is *Paeonia lactiflora* Pall., consisting of monoterpenoids, triterpenoids, flavonoids, phenols and tannins. Its main bioavailable compounds consist of paeoniflorin, pentagalloylglucose, gallic acid, albiflorin and benzoic acid.[94]

In a rat cerebral artery occlusion model, paeoniflorin has shown to be neuroprotective. Via activation of adenosine A1 receptor, it reduces infarct volume and neurological impairment.[95] Furthermore, a study in which the carotid artery of rats was also occluded indicated reduction in ED1, IL-1beta, TNF-α and ICAM-1 of micro-vessels which may explain subsequent decreases in apoptosis.[96] In LPS-stimulated mice, paeoniflorin reduces TNF-α and IL-1β release.[97] Paeoniflorin may also be beneficial for improving muscle strength and function post-stroke, increasing expression of nuclear factor-YA (NF-YA) and molecules mitigating impairment from muscular atrophy.[98]

In an hypoxic/ischaemic *in vitro* model, via inhibition of oxidative stress and targeting mitochondrial permeability transition pores, gallic acid can modulate mitochondrial dysfunction.[99] When mice are fed high-fat diets, gallic acid shows hypolipidemic activity, indicating its potential as a preventer of stroke.[100] Exploring this hypolipidemic activity, gallic acid administered to rats on similar diets results in decreased serum triglyceride, phospholipids, total cholesterol and LDL-cholesterol.[101] Such decreases to triglyceride and LDL cholesterol plasma can reduce blood pressure and thus the risk of stroke.[100]

Experimentally, albiflorin has similar anti-inflammatory effects to paeoniflorin, with comparative studies showing it inhibits NO, PGE2, TNF-α and IL-6, as well as reducing expression of COX-2.[102]

Paeonal has both neuroprotective and anti-inflammatory activity which may be therapeutic for stroke. In rat carotid and cerebral artery occlusion models, via reductions to micoglia activation, lucigenin-chemiluminescence (CL) counts, ED1 and IL-1β immunoreactive cells, paeonal administration reduces infarct size and improves neurological scores.[103] In hippocampal slice culture and rat brain primary microglial cells, paeonal blocks LPS-related hippocampal death and inhibits NO and IL-1β release from microglial cells.[104]

Experimental Studies on *sang zhi*

The botanical source of *sang zhi* 桑枝 is *Morus alba* L. and consists largely of mulberroside A, oxyresveratrol, resveratrol, ramulus mori polysaccharides maclurin, rutin, isoquercitrin, morin and nojirimycin.[105,106]

From *sang zhi*, ramulus mori polysaccharide extract has evidence of potential hypoglycaemic, anti-inflammatory and antiplatelet activity.[107–109] In fasting rats and mice, the extract lowers blood glucose concentration.[110] Hypoglycaemic benefits could reduce diabetes risk and subsequently risk of stroke complications. In the streptozotocin (STZ)-induced diabetic mouse model, in addition to hypoglycaemic effects, pancreatic tissue shows decreased expression of TNF-α, IL-8, IL-6 and COX-2.[111] Subsequent experiments from the same model confirm anti-inflammatory activity of the extract, increasing Bcl-2 expression, reducing pancreatic tissue Bax protein levels and downregulating expression of p-JNK, p-p38 and cleaved-caspase-3.[112] In an *in vivo* rat model of carotid arterial thrombosis, extracts have shown antiplatelet activity with potential for stroke prevention, inhibiting platelet aggregation and subsequently preventing thrombosis.[113]

In mouse pain and inflammatory models, cis-mulberroside A has been evidenced to be an antioxidant, reducing the production of NO and expression of iNOS.[114]

Also of interest for stroke are morin and morusin. Although not only specific to *Ramulus mori*, review of morin indicates it has antioxidant, antidiabetic, anti-inflammatory, antitumoral, antihypertensive, antibacterial, hypouricemic and neuroprotective effects.[115] In tumour-effected mice, anti-inflammatory activity of morusin sees it scavenge free radicals, inhibit COX-1 generation of superoxide anion, and modulate caspase-3 and NF-κB genes.[116]

Experimental Studies on *tao ren*

Sourced from the kernel of *Prunus persica* (L.) Batsch or *Prunus davidiana* (Carr.) Franch., tao ren 桃仁 predominantly contains phenols, flavonoids and carotenoids.[117] There is variation in content between pulp, peel and seed, with gallic acid, protocatechuic acid, protocatechualdehyde, chlorogenic acid, p-coumaric acid and ferulic acid the main constituents of pulp and amygdalin a major component of seeds.[117,118]

Pharmacological inhibition and genetic targeting of myostatin have implicated it for treatment of muscular disease, and follistatin is an autocrine glycoprotein with a strong ability to antagonize myostatin.[119] In skeletal muscle, extracts of tao ren increase expression of follistatin mRNA and stimulates growth of skeletal muscle cell lines.[120] Such activity may have post-stroke benefits in patients with muscle wasting by increasing skeletal muscle mass and strength.[121,122] It has been proposed that the biological activity of the extract is due to its content of amygdalin.[120] In rat dopaminergic PC12 cells, amygdalin induces activation of ERK1/2 to support growth and differentiation of cells.[123] Amygdalin also shows platelet inhibitory activity for preventing stroke, without risk to blood viscosity, as it decreases prothombin time, reduces platelet aggregation and protects vascular endothelial cells.[124]

Summary of Pharmacological Actions of the Common Herbs

Extracts of herbal medicine and individual herbal compounds have experimentally shown therapeutic bioactivity relevant to stroke. Such activity is largely neuroprotective, anticoagulant, antioxidant/anti-inflammatory and hypotensive, with also some regenerative activity of cells relevant to stroke.

Neuroprotective and cytoprotective activity has been evidenced through the ability of some compounds to permeate the BBB and inhibit cellular apoptosis to reduce neurophysiological damage from stoke and to protect cognition.

Anticoagulant and antiplatelet activity is evidenced by reduced thrombus size in various experimental models and prolonged clotting, with potential to prevent clot formation and physical blockage of vessels in the brain which can cause stroke.

Hypotensive activity has been evidenced by reduced blood pressure from decreased total cholesterol and triglycerides, which can assist to prevent cardiovascular damage leading to stroke.

Anti-inflammatory and antioxidant activity has shown to reduce many of the inflammatory factors associated with tissue injury, which has potential to limit cellular damage caused by a stroke and its physiological impacts.

There is some evidence of tissue regenerative activity, which might assist in synthesising muscular tissue lost to wasting post-stroke, and improving muscular strength and function in affected regions. Neurogenesis has also been evidenced in some parts of the brain, such as the hippocampus, which could benefit neural recovery and function post-stroke by improving nerve conduction.

References

1. Hong B, Wang Z, Xu T, *et al.* (2015) Matrix solid-phase dispersion extraction followed by high performance liquid chromatography-diode array detection and ultra performance liquid chromatography-quadrupole-time of flight-mass spectrometer method for the determination of the main compounds from Carthamus tinctorius L. (Hong-hua). *J Pharm Biomed Anal* **107**: 464–472.

2. Zhou X, Tang L, Xu Y, *et al.* (2014) Towards a better understanding of medicinal uses of Carthamus tinctorius L. in traditional Chinese medicine: A phytochemical and pharmacological review. *J Ethnopharmacol* **151**(1): 27–43.

3. Wang Y, Chen P, Tang C, *et al.* (2014) Antinociceptive and anti-inflammatory activities of extract and two isolated flavonoids of Carthamus tinctorius L. *J Ethnopharmacol* **151**(2): 944–950.

4. Jun MS, Ha YM, Kim HS, *et al.* (2011) Anti-inflammatory action of methanol extract of Carthamus tinctorius L. involves in hemeoxygenase-1 induction. *J Ethnopharmacol* **133**(2): 524–530.

5. Hiramatsu M, Takahashi T, Komatsu M, *et al.* (2009) Antioxidant and neuroprotective activities of Mogami-benibana (safflower, Carthamus tinctorius L.). *Neurochem Res* **34**(4): 795–805.

6. Li Y, Wang N. (2010) Antithrombotic effects of Danggui, Honghua and potential drug interaction with clopidogrel. *J Ethnopharmacol* **128**(3): 623–628.

7. Wan LH, Chen J, Li L, *et al.* (2011) Protective effects of Carthamus tinctorius injection on isoprenaline-induced myocardial injury in rats. *Pharm Biol* **49**(11): 1204–1209.

8. Nobakht M, Fattahi M, Hoormand M, *et al.* (2000) A study on the teratogenic and cytotoxic effects of safflower extract. *J Ethnopharmacol* **73**(3): 453–459.

9. Li HX, Han SY, Wang XW, *et al.* (2009) Effect of the carthamins yellow from Carthamus tinctorius L. on hemorheological disorders of blood stasis in rats. *Food Chem Toxicol* **47**(8): 1797–1802.

10. Wang CC, Choy CS, Liu YH, *et al.* (2011) Protective effect of dried safflower petal aqueous extract and its main constituent, carthamus yellow, against lipopolysaccharide-induced inflammation in RAW264.7 macrophages. *J Sci Food Agric* **91**(2): 218–225.

11. Ji DB, Zhu MC, Zhu B, *et al.* (2008) Hydroxysafflor yellow A enhances survival of vascular endothelial cells under hypoxia via upregulation of the HIF-1 alpha-VEGF pathway and regulation of Bcl-2/Bax. *J Cardiovasc Pharmacol* **52**(2): 191–202.

12. Zhu HB, Wang ZH, Tian JW, *et al.* (2005) Protective effect of hydroxysafflor yellow A on experimental cerebral ischemia in rats [article in Chinese]. *Yao xue xue bao* — Acta pharmaceutica Sinica] **40**(12): 1144–1146.

13. Pan Y, Zheng DY, Liu SM, *et al.* (2012) Hydroxysafflor yellow A attenuates lymphostatic encephalopathy-induced brain injury in rats. *Phytother Res* **26**(10): 1500–1506.

14. Zang BX, Jin M, Si N, *et al.* (2002) Antagonistic effect of hydroxysafflor yellow A on the platelet activating factor receptor [article in Chinese]. *Yao xue xue bao* — Acta pharmaceutica Sinica **37**(9): 696–699.

15. Hotta Y, Nagatsu A, Liu W, *et al.* (2002) Protective effects of antioxidative serotonin derivatives isolated from safflower against postischemic myocardial dysfunction. *Mol Cell Biochem* **238**(1–2): 151–162.

16. Yadava RN, Chakravarti N. (2008) Anti-inflammatory activity of a new triterpenoid saponin from Carthamus tinctorius L. *J Enzyme Inhib Med Chem* **23**(4): 543–548.

17. Yang J, Chen LH, Zhang Q, *et al.* (2007) Quality assessment of cortex cinnamomi by HPLC chemical fingerprint, principle component analysis and cluster analysis. *J Sep Sci* **30**(9): 1276–1283.
18. He ZD, Qiao CF, Han QB, *et al.* (2005) Authentication and quantitative analysis on the chemical profile of cassia bark (cortex cinnamomi) by high-pressure liquid chromatography. *J Agric Food Chem* **53**(7): 2424–2428.
19. Takasao N, Tsuji-Naito K, Ishikura S, *et al.* (2012) Cinnamon extract promotes type I collagen biosynthesis via activation of IGF-I signaling in human dermal fibroblasts. *J Agric Food Chem* **60**(5): 1193–1200.
20. Brosnan JT, Brosnan ME. (2007) Creatine: Endogenous metabolite, dietary, and therapeutic supplement. *Annu Rev Nutr* **27**: 241–261.
21. Zdzieblik D, Oesser S, Baumstark MW, *et al.* (2015) Collagen peptide supplementation in combination with resistance training improves body composition and increases muscle strength in elderly sarcopenic men: A randomised controlled trial. *Br J Nutr* **114**(8): 1237–1245.
22. Lee HS, Kim BS, Kim MK. (2002) Suppression effect of Cinnamomum cassia bark-derived component on nitric oxide synthase. *J Agric Food Chem* **50**(26): 7700–7703.
23. Zhao J, Zhang X, Dong L, *et al.* (2015) Cinnamaldehyde inhibits inflammation and brain damage in a mouse model of permanent cerebral ischaemia. *Br J Pharmacol* **172**(20): 5009–5023.
24. Chen YF, Wang YW, Huang WS, *et al.* (2016) Trans-cinnamaldehyde, an essential oil in cinnamon powder, ameliorates cerebral ischemia-induced brain injury via inhibition of neuroinflammation through Attenuation of iNOS, COX-2 expression and NFkappa-B signaling pathway. *Neuromol Med* **18**(3): 322–333.
25. Silva CR, Oliveira SM, Rossato MF, *et al.* (2011) The involvement of TRPA1 channel activation in the inflammatory response evoked by topical application of cinnamaldehyde to mice. *Life Sci* **88**(25–26): 1077–1087.
26. Olsen RV, Andersen HH, Moller HG, *et al.* (2014) Somatosensory and vasomotor manifestations of individual and combined stimulation of TRPM8 and TRPA1 using topical L-menthol and trans-cinnamaldehyde in healthy volunteers. *Eur J Pain* **18**(9): 1333–1342.
27. Chao WW, Lin BF. (2011) Bioactivities of major constituents isolated from Angelica sinensis (*Danggui*). *Chin Med* **6**: 29.
28. Li Y, Wang SW, Tu HH, Cao W. (2013) Simultaneous quantification of six main active constituents in Chinese Angelica by high-performance

liquid chromatography with photodiode array detector. *Pharmacogn Mag* **9**(34): 114–119.

29. Xin J, Zhang J, Yang Y, *et al.* (2013) Radix Angelica Sinensis that contains the component Z-ligustilide promotes adult neurogenesis to mediate recovery from cognitive impairment. *Curr Neurovasc Res* **10**(4): 304–315.

30. Cheng CY, Ho TY, Lee EJ, *et al.* (2008) Ferulic acid reduces cerebral infarct through its antioxidative and anti-inflammatory effects following transient focal cerebral ischemia in rats. *Am J Chin Med* **36**(6): 1105–1119.

31. Cheng CY, Su SY, Tang NY, *et al.* (2008) Ferulic acid provides neuroprotection against oxidative stress-related apoptosis after cerebral ischemia/reperfusion injury by inhibiting ICAM-1 mRNA expression in rats. *Brain Res* **1209**: 136–150.

32. Zhang L, Wang H, Wang T, *et al.* (2015) Ferulic acid ameliorates nerve injury induced by cerebral ischemia in rats. *Exp Ther Med* **9**(3): 972–976.

33. Lee SC, Tsai CC, Yao CH, *et al.* (2013) Ferulic acid enhances peripheral nerve regeneration across long gaps. *Evid Based Complement Alternat Med* **2013**: 876327.

34. Ardiansyah, Ohsaki Y, Shirakawa H, *et al.* (2008) Novel effects of a single administration of ferulic acid on the regulation of blood pressure and the hepatic lipid metabolic profile in stroke-prone spontaneously hypertensive rats. *J Agric Food Chem* **56**(8): 2825–2830.

35. Guo J, Shang EX, Duan JA, *et al.* (2011) Determination of ligustilide in the brains of freely moving rats using microdialysis coupled with ultra performance liquid chromatography/mass spectrometry. *Fitoterapia* **82**(3): 441–445.

36. Kuang X, Du JR, Liu YX, *et al.* (2008) Postischemic administration of Z-ligustilide ameliorates cognitive dysfunction and brain damage induced by permanent forebrain ischemia in rats. *Pharmacol Biochem Behav* **88**(3): 213–221.

37. Peng HY, Du JR, Zhang GY, *et al.* (2007) Neuroprotective effect of Z-ligustilide against permanent focal ischemic damage in rats. *Biol Pharm Bull* **30**(2): 309–312.

38. Chen D, Tang J, Khatibi NH, *et al.* (2011) Treatment with Z-ligustilide, a component of Angelica sinensis, reduces brain injury after a subarachnoid hemorrhage in rats. *J Pharmacol Exp Ther* **337**(3): 663–672.

39. Feng Z, Lu Y, Wu X, *et al.* (2012) Ligustilide alleviates brain damage and improves cognitive function in rats of chronic cerebral hypoperfusion. *J Ethnopharmacol* **144**(2): 313–321.
40. Chi K, Fu RH, Huang YC, *et al.* (2016) Therapeutic effect of ligustilide-stimulated adipose-derived stem cells in a mouse thromboembolic stroke model. *Cell Transplant* **25**(5): 899–912.
41. Mimura Y, Kobayashi S, Naitoh T, *et al.* (1995) The structure-activity relationship between synthetic butylidenephthalide derivatives regarding the competence and progression of inhibition in primary cultures proliferation of mouse aorta smooth muscle cells. *Biol Pharm Bull* **18**(9): 1203–1206.
42. Teng CM, Chen WY, Ko WC, Ouyang CH. (1987) Antiplatelet effect of butylidenephthalide. *Biochim Biophys Acta* **924**(3): 375–382.
43. Nam KN, Kim KP, Cho KH, *et al.* (2013) Prevention of inflammation-mediated neurotoxicity by butylidenephthalide and its role in microglial activation. *Cell Biochem Funct* **31**(8): 707–712.
44. Lei H, Zhao CY, Liu DM, *et al.* (2014) l-3-n-butylphthalide attenuates beta-amyloid-induced toxicity in neuroblastoma SH-SY5Y cells through regulating mitochondrion-mediated apoptosis and MAPK signaling. *J Asian Nat Prod Res* **16**(8): 854–864.
45. He CY, Wang S, Feng Y, *et al.* (2012) Pharmacokinetics, tissue distribution and metabolism of senkyunolide I, a major bioactive component in Ligusticum chuanxiong Hort. (Umbelliferae). *J Ethnopharmacol* **142**(3): 706–713.
46. Hu PY, Liu D, Zheng Q, *et al.* (2016) Elucidation of transport mechanism of paeoniflorin and the influence of ligustilide, senkyunolide I and senkyunolide a on paeoniflorin transport through Mdck-Mdr1 cells as blood-brain barrier *in vitro* model. *Molecules* **21**(3): 300.
47. Hu Y, Duan M, Liang S, *et al.* (2015) Senkyunolide I protects rat brain against focal cerebral ischemia-reperfusion injury by up-regulating p-Erk1/2, Nrf2/HO-1 and inhibiting caspase 3. *Brain Res* **1605**: 39–48.
48. Zhao YX, Ding MY, Liu DL. (2005) Phenolic acids analysis in ligusticum chuanxiong using HPLC. *J Chromatogr Sci* **43**(8): 389–393.
49. Liu JL, Zheng SL, Fan QJ, *et al.* (2014) Optimization of high-pressure ultrasonic-assisted simultaneous extraction of six major constituents from Ligusticum chuanxiong rhizome using response surface methodology. *Molecules* **19**(2): 1887–1911.

50. Or TC, Yang CL, Law AH, *et al.* (2011) Isolation and identification of anti-inflammatory constituents from Ligusticum chuanxiong and their underlying mechanisms of action on microglia. *Neuropharmacology* **60**(6): 823–831.

51. Liao SL, Kao TK, Chen WY, *et al.* (2004) Tetramethylpyrazine reduces ischemic brain injury in rats. *Neurosci Lett* **372**(1–2): 40–45.

52. Yan Y, Zhao J, Cao C, *et al.* (2014) Tetramethylpyrazine promotes SH-SY5Y cell differentiation into neurons through epigenetic regulation of Topoisomerase IIbeta. *Neuroscience* **278**: 179–193.

53. Tian Y, Liu Y, Chen X, *et al.* (2010) Tetramethylpyrazine promotes proliferation and differentiation of neural stem cells from rat brain in hypoxic condition via mitogen-activated protein kinases pathway *in vitro. Neurosci Lett* **474**(1): 26–31.

54. Kong X, Zhong M, Su X, *et al.* (2016) Tetramethylpyrazine promotes migration of neural precursor cells via activating the phosphatidylinositol 3-kinase pathway. *Mol Neurobiol* **53**(9): 6526–6539 .

55. Zhang M, Gao F, Teng F, Zhang C. (2014) Tetramethylpyrazine promotes the proliferation and migration of brain endothelial cells. *Mol Med Rep* **10**(1): 29–32.

56. Cai X, Chen Z, Pan X, *et al.* (2014) Inhibition of angiogenesis, fibrosis and thrombosis by tetramethylpyrazine: Mechanisms contributing to the SDF-1/CXCR4 axis. *PloS one* **9**(2): e88176.

57. Lin F, Zhang C, Chen X, *et al.* (2015) Chrysophanol affords neuroprotection against microglial activation and free radical-mediated oxidative damage in BV2 murine microglia. *Int J Clin Exp Med* **8**(3): 3447–3455.

58. *Zhong Hua Ben Cao: Jing Xuan Ben* [Chinese Materia Medica: abridged version] (1998) Shanghai Scientific and Technical Publishers, Shanghai.

59. Shi JG, Wang HQ, Wang M, Zhu Y. (1995) Two pyridine-2,6(1H,3H)-dione alkaloids from Speranskia tuberculata. *Phytochemistry* **40**(4): 1299–1302.

60. Shi JG, Wang HQ, Wang M, *et al.* (2000) Polyoxygenated bipyridine, pyrrolylpyridine, and bipyrrole alkaloids from Speranskia tuberculata. *J Nat Prod* **63**(6): 782–786.

61. Chua LS. (2016) Untargeted MS-based small metabolite identification from the plant leaves and stems of Impatiens balsamina. *Plant Physiol Biochem* **106**: 16–22.

62. Sakunphueak A, Panichayupakaranant P. (2010) Simultaneous determination of three naphthoquinones in the leaves of Impatiens balsamina L. by reversed-phase high-performance liquid chromatography. *Phytochem Anal* **21**(5): 444–450.

63. Devi KP, Malar DS, Nabavi SF, *et al.* (2015) Kaempferol and inflammation: From chemistry to medicine. *Pharmacol Res* **99**: 1–10.

64. Crespo I, Garcia-Mediavilla MV, Gutierrez B, *et al.* (2008) A comparison of the effects of kaempferol and quercetin on cytokine-induced pro-inflammatory status of cultured human endothelial cells. *Br J Nutr* **100**(5): 968–976.

65. Oku H, Ishiguro K. (2002) Cyclooxygenase-2 inhibitory 1,4-naphthoquinones from Impatiens balsamina L. *Biol Pharm Bull* **25**(5): 658–660.

66. Fang X, Wang J, Yu X, *et al.* (2010) Optimization of microwave-assisted extraction followed by RP-HPLC for the simultaneous determination of oleanolic acid and ursolic acid in the fruits of Chaenomeles sinensis. *J Sep Sci* **33**(8): 1147–1155.

67. Du H, Wu J, Li H, *et al.* (2013) Polyphenols and triterpenes from Chaenomeles fruits: Chemical analysis and antioxidant activities assessment. *Food Chem* **141**(4): 4260–4268.

68. Kylli P, Nohynek L, Puupponen-Pimia R, *et al.* (2011) Lingonberry (Vaccinium vitis-idaea) and European cranberry (Vaccinium microcarpon) proanthocyanidins: Isolation, identification and bioactivities. *J Agric Food Chem* **59**(7): 3373–3384.

69. Rasmussen SE, Frederiksen H, Struntze Krogholm K, Poulsen L. (2005) Dietary proanthocyanidins: Occurrence, dietary intake, bioavailability and protection against cardiovascular disease. *Mol Nutr Food Res* **49**(2): 159–174.

70. Ma B, Wang J, Tong J, *et al.* (2016) Protective effects of Chaenomeles thibetica extract against carbon tetrachloride-induced damage via the MAPK/Nrf2 pathway. *Food Funct* **7**(3): 1492–1500.

71. Strugala P, Cyboran-Mikolajczyk S, Dudra A, *et al.* (2016) Biological activity of Japanese quince extract and its interactions with lipids, erythrocyte membrane, and human albumin. *J Membr Biol* **249**(3): 393–410.

72. Zhu Q, Liao C, Liu Y, *et al.* (2012) Ethanolic extract and water-soluble polysaccharide from Chaenomeles speciosa fruit modulate lipopolysaccharide-induced nitric oxide production in RAW264.7 macrophage cells. *J Ethnopharmacol* **144**(2): 441–447.

73. Dai M, Wei W, Shen YX, Zheng YQ. (2003) Glucosides of Chaenomeles speciosa remit rat adjuvant arthritis by inhibiting synoviocyte activities. *Acta Pharmacol Sin* **24**(11): 1161–1166.

74. Chen Q, Wei W. (2003) Effects and mechanisms of glucosides of Chaenomeles speciosa on collagen-induced arthritis in rats. *Int Immunopharmacol* **3**(4): 593–608.

75. Xie X, Zou G, Li C. (2015) Antitumor and immunomodulatory activities of a water-soluble polysaccharide from Chaenomeles speciosa. *Carbohydr Polym* **132**: 323–329.

76. Zhang L, Cheng YX, Liu AL, *et al.* (2010) Antioxidant, anti-inflammatory and anti-influenza properties of components from *Chaenomeles speciosa*. *Molecules* **15**(11): 8507–8517.

77. Cho SO, Ban JY, Kim JY, *et al.* (2009) Anti-ischemic activities of aralia cordata and its active component, oleanolic acid. *Arch Pharm Res* **32**(6): 923–932.

78. Rong ZT, Gong XJ, Sun HB, *et al.* (2011) Protective effects of oleanolic acid on cerebral ischemic damage *in vivo* and $H(2)O(2)$-induced injury *in vitro*. *Pharm Biol* **49**(1): 78–85.

79. Li L, Zhang X, Cui L, *et al.* (2013) Ursolic acid promotes the neuroprotection by activating Nrf2 pathway after cerebral ischemia in mice. *Brain Res* **1497**: 32–39.

80. Kim HY, Choi HR, Lee YJ, *et al.* (2014) Accentuation of ursolic acid on muscarinic receptor-induced ANP secretion in beating rabbit atria. *Life Sci* **94**(2): 145–150.

81. Park YJ, Thwe AA, Li X, *et al.* (2015) Triterpene and flavonoid biosynthesis and metabolic profiling of hairy roots, adventitious roots, and seedling roots of astragalus membranaceus. *J Agric Food Chem* **63**(40): 8862–8869.

82. Chen CC, Lee HC, Chang JH, *et al.* (2012) Chinese herb astragalus membranaceus enhances recovery of hemorrhagic stroke: Double-blind, placebo-controlled, randomized study. *Evid Based Complement Alternat Med* **2012**: 708452.

83. Cai J, Pan R, Jia X, *et al.* (2014) The combination of astragalus membranaceus and ligustrazine ameliorates micro-haemorrhage by maintaining blood-brain barrier integrity in cerebrally ischaemic rats. *J Ethnopharmacol* **158**(Pt A): 301–309.

84. Li M, Ma RN, Li LH, *et al.* (2013) Astragaloside IV reduces cerebral edema post-ischemia/reperfusion correlating the suppression of MMP-9 and AQP4. *Eur J Pharmacol* **715**(1–3): 189–195.

85. Ren S, Zhang H, Mu Y, *et al.* (2013) Pharmacological effects of Astragaloside IV: A literature review. *J Tradit Chin Med* **33**(3): 413–416.

86. Qu YZ, Li M, Zhao YL, *et al.* (2009) Astragaloside IV attenuates cerebral ischemia-reperfusion-induced increase in permeability of the blood-brain barrier in rats. *Eur J Pharmacol* **606**(1–3): 137–141.

87. Shao A, Guo S, Tu S, *et al.* (2014) Astragaloside IV alleviates early brain injury following experimental subarachnoid hemorrhage in rats. *Int J Med Sci* **11**(10): 1073–1081.

88. Zhang WD, Zhang C, Liu RH, *et al.* (2006) Preclinical pharmacokinetics and tissue distribution of a natural cardioprotective agent astragaloside IV in rats and dogs. *Life Sci* **79**(8): 808–815.

89. Gao J, Liu ZJ, Chen T, Zhao D. (2014) Pharmaceutical properties of calycosin, the major bioactive isoflavonoid in the dry root extract of Radix astragali. *Pharm Biol* **52**(9): 1217–1222.

90. Guo C, Tong L, Xi M, *et al.* (2012) Neuroprotective effect of calycosin on cerebral ischemia and reperfusion injury in rats. *J Ethnopharmacol* **144**(3): 768–774.

91. Wang Y, Dong X, Li Z, *et al.* (2014) Downregulated RASD1 and upregulated miR-375 are involved in protective effects of calycosin on cerebral ischemia/reperfusion rats. *J Neurol Sci* **339**(1–2): 144–148.

92. Fu S, Gu Y, Jiang JQ, *et al.* (2014) Calycosin-7-O-beta-D-glucoside regulates nitric oxide/caveolin-1/matrix metalloproteinases pathway and protects blood-brain barrier integrity in experimental cerebral ischemia-reperfusion injury. *J Ethnopharmacol* **155**(1): 692–701.

93. Junqing G, Tao C, Huigen J, *et al.* (2015) Effect of calycosin on left ventricular ejection fraction and angiogenesis in rat models with myocardial infarction. *J Tradit Chin Med* **35**(2): 160–167.

94. Parker S, May B, Zhang C, *et al.* (2016) A pharmacological review of bioactive constituents of Paeonia lactiflora Pallas and Paeonia veitchii Lynch. *Phytother Res* **30**(9): 1445–1473.

95. Liu DZ, Xie KQ, Ji XQ, *et al.* (2005) Neuroprotective effect of paeoniflorin on cerebral ischemic rat by activating adenosine A1 receptor in a manner different from its classical agonists. *Br J Pharmacol* **146**(4): 604–611.

96. Tang NY, Liu CH, Hsieh CT, Hsieh CL. (2010) The anti-inflammatory effect of paeoniflorin on cerebral infarction induced by ischemia-reperfusion injury in Sprague-Dawley rats. *Am J Chin Med* **38**(1): 51–64.

97. Cao W, Zhang W, Liu J, *et al.* (2011) Paeoniflorin improves survival in LPS-challenged mice through the suppression of TNF-alpha and IL-1beta release and augmentation of IL-10 production. *Int Immunopharmacol* **11**(2): 172–178.

98. Tohnai G, Adachi H, Katsuno M, *et al.* (2014) Paeoniflorin eliminates a mutant AR via NF-YA-dependent proteolysis in spinal and bulbar muscular atrophy. *Hum Mol Genet* **23**(13): 3552–3565.

99. Sun J, Li YZ, Ding YH, *et al.* (2014) Neuroprotective effects of gallic acid against hypoxia/reoxygenation-induced mitochondrial dysfunctions *in vitro* and cerebral ischemia/reperfusion injury *in vivo. Brain Res* **1589**: 126–139.

100. Jang A, Srinivasan P, Lee NY, *et al.* (2008) Comparison of hypolipidemic activity of synthetic gallic acid-linoleic acid ester with mixture of gallic acid and linoleic acid, gallic acid, and linoleic acid on high-fat diet induced obesity in C57BL/6 Cr Slc mice. *Chem Biol Interact* **174**(2):109–117.

101. Hsu CL, Yen GC. (2007) Effect of gallic acid on high fat diet-induced dyslipidaemia, hepatosteatosis and oxidative stress in rats. *Br J Nutr* **98**(4): 727–735.

102. Wang QS, Gao T, Cui YL, *et al.* (2014) Comparative studies of paeoniflorin and albiflorin from Paeonia lactiflora on anti-inflammatory activities. *Pharm Biol* **52**(9): 1189–1195.

103. Hsieh CL, Cheng CY, Tsai TH, *et al.* (2006) Paeonol reduced cerebral infarction involving the superoxide anion and microglia activation in ischemia-reperfusion injured rats. *J Ethnopharmacol* **106**(2): 208–215.

104. Nam K, Woo B, Moon S, *et al.* (2013) Paeonol attenuates inflammation-mediated neurotoxicity and microglial activation. *Neural Regen Res* **8**(18): 1637–1643.

105. Zhou J, Li S, Wang W, *et al.* (2013) Variations in the levels of mulberroside A, oxyresveratrol, and resveratrol in mulberries in different seasons and during growth. *Sci World J* **2013**: 380692.

106. Chang L, Juang L, Wang B, *et al.* (2011) Antioxidant and antityrosinase activity of mulberry (Morus alba L.) twigs and root bark. *Food Chem Toxicol* **49**(4): 785–790.

107. Liu Y, Shen Z, Chen Z, *et al.* (2010) The use of the effective section of alkaloids from ramulus mori for preparation of a hypoglycemig agent. EP application (EP2255822A1).

108. The use of the effective section of alkaloids from ramulus mori for preparation of a hypoglycemic agent. European Patent Office (patent No. EP2255822A1). 2010. Available from https://patents.google.com/patent/EP2255822A1.

109. Liu Y, Shen Z, Chen Z, *et al.* (2015) Use of the effective fraction of alkaloids from mulberry twig in preparing hypoglycemic agents. Patnet (US9066960B2). United States.

110. Ye F, Shen Z, Xie M. (2002) Alpha-glucosidase inhibition from a Chinese medical herb (Ramulus mori) in normal and diabetic rats and mice. *Phytomedicine* **9**(2): 161–166.

111. Guo C, Li R, Zheng N, *et al.* (2013) Anti-diabetic effect of ramulus mori polysaccharides, isolated from Morus alba L., on STZ-diabetic mice through blocking inflammatory response and attenuating oxidative stress. *Int Immunopharmacol* **16**(1): 93–99.

112. Xu L, Yang F, Wang J, *et al.* (2015) Anti-diabetic effect mediated by Ramulus mori polysaccharides. *Carbohydr Polym* **117**: 63–69.

113. Lee J, Kwon G, Park J, *et al.* (2016) An ethanol extract of Ramulus mori improves blood circulation by inhibiting platelet aggregation. *Biosci Biotechnol Biochem* **80**(7): 1410–1415.

114. Zhang Z, Shi L. (2010) Anti-inflammatory and analgesic properties of cis-mulberroside A from Ramulus mori. *Fitoterapia* **81**(3): 214–218.

115. Caselli A, Cirri P, Santi A, Paoli P. (2016) Morin: A promising natural drug. *Curr Med Chem* **23**(8): 774–791.

116. Wan LZ, Ma B, Zhang YQ. (2014) Preparation of morusin from Ramulus mori and its effects on mice with transplanted H22 hepatocarcinoma. *Biofactors* **40**(6): 636–645.

117. Loizzo MR, Pacetti D, Lucci P, *et al.* (2015) Prunus persica var. platycarpa (Tabacchiera Peach): Bioactive compounds and antioxidant activity of pulp, peel and seed ethanolic extracts. *Plant Foods Hum Nutr* **70**(3): 331–337.

118. Tanaka R, Nitta A, Nagatsu A. (2014) Application of a quantitative 1H-NMR method for the determination of amygdalin in Persicae semen, Armeniacae semen, and Mume fructus. *J Nat Med* **68**(1): 225–230.

119. Rodino-Klapac LR, Haidet AM, Kota J, *et al.* (2009) Inhibition of myostatin with emphasis on follistatin as a therapy for muscle disease. *Muscle Nerve* **39**(3): 283–296.

120. Yang C, Li X, Rong J. (2014) Amygdalin isolated from Semen Persicae (*tao ren*) extracts induces the expression of follistatin in HepG2 and C2C12 cell lines. *Chin Med* **9**: 23.

121. Siriett V, Salerno MS, Berry C, *et al.* (2007) Antagonism of myostatin enhances muscle regeneration during sarcopenia. *Mol Ther* **15**(8): 1463–1470.

122. Whittemore LA, Song K, Li X, *et al.* (2003) Inhibition of myostatin in adult mice increases skeletal muscle mass and strength. *Biochem Biophys Res Commun* **300**(4): 965–971.

123. Yang C, Zhao J, Cheng Y, *et al.* (2014) Bioactivity-guided fractionation identifies amygdalin as a potent neurotrophic agent from herbal medicine Semen Persicae extract. *Biomed Res Int* **2014**: 306857.

124. Liu L, Duan JA, Tang Y, *et al.* (2012) *Tao ren-hong hua* herb pair and its main components promoting blood circulation through influencing on hemorheology, plasma coagulation and platelet aggregation. *J Ethnopharmacol* **139**(2): 381–387.

7

Clinical Evidence for Acupuncture and Related Therapies

OVERVIEW

Acupuncture therapies are commonly researched in clinical studies for post-stroke shoulder complications involving shoulder subluxation, shoulder pain and shoulder-hand syndrome. Extensive searches of nine electronic databases identified over 37,000 citations for the condition. One hundred and one randomised controlled trials, three controlled clinical trials and 31 non-controlled studies were included in this chapter. The results showed that the evidence of acupuncture therapies was promising, particularly for patients' motor function, pain and activities of daily living.

Introduction

Acupuncture is a common technique to treat disease by correcting imbalances and restoring health. Methods of stimulating acupuncture points include:

- Acupuncture: Insertion of an acupuncture needle into acupuncture points;
- Acupressure: Application of pressure to acupuncture points;
- Moxibustion: Burning of a herb (usually *ai ye* 艾叶, *Artemesia vulgaris* L.) close to, or on, the skin to induce a warming sensation;
- Electroacupuncture: Electric stimulation of the needle following insertion;

- Scalp acupuncture 头皮针: Acupuncture micro-system at the specific lines located on the scalp;
- Wrist-ankle acupuncture 腕踝针: Acupuncture micro-system at six points located on wrist and ankle;
- Floating acupuncture 浮针: Acupuncture at subcutaneous superficial fascia rather than traditional acupuncture points.

Whilst all of these therapies have ancient roots, several have emerged as new techniques in the last century. For example, electroacupuncture is a technique that combines acupuncture with electric stimulation; wrist-ankle acupuncture 腕踝针 and scalp acupuncture 头皮针 was generated based on the reflexology theory, while the floating acupuncture 浮针 method is a combination of traditional acupuncture therapy and modern medicine anatomy knowledge.

Previous Systematic Reviews

The efficacy and safety of acupuncture-related therapies for post-stroke shoulder complications have been systematically reviewed by one publication published in English[1] and five published in Chinese.[2–6]

Shoulder Pain

Lee (2012)[1] reviewed seven randomised control trials (RCTs) of acupuncture for post-stroke shoulder pain. All of the included studies were conducted in China and published in Chinese. Of these studies, three compared the combination of acupuncture and rehabilitation to rehabilitation alone, one compared this combination to drug therapy, one compared this combination to acupuncture alone, one compared acupuncture plus exercise to drug therapy plus exercise, and another one compared the combination of electroacupuncture and transcutaneous electrical nerve stimulation (TENS) to electroacupuncture alone. Based on the Modified Jadad Scores and the Cochrane Back Review Group Criteria List for Methodological

Quality Assessment of RCTs, the methodological quality of included RCTs was assessed as 'moderate' on average. Outcomes reported by all included RCTs varied, with the common ones being visual analogue scale (VAS), reported by five RCTs; and Fugl-Meyer Assessment (FMA) and range of motion (ROM) (each of which was reported by three RCTs). Meta-analysis was not performed due to the diversity of interventions, although the authors stated that their review provided suggestive evidence for the effectiveness of acupuncture in treating shoulder pain after stroke.

Nie (2012)[2] systematically reviewed 12 RCTs, all of which were published in Chinese. All RCTs compared the combination of acupuncture therapies and rehabilitation to rehabilitation alone, except one which compared the combination of acupuncture and Chinese herbal medicine (CHM) to CHM alone. Acupuncture therapies included body acupuncture (eight studies), and scalp acupuncture, abdomen acupuncture, electroacupuncture and moxibustion therapy (one study of each). Using Jadad Scores to assess the methodological quality, all RCTs were assessed as low quality. Outcomes used for meta-analyses were pain score, FMA, ROM, Barthel Index (BI) and effective rate. Meta-analysis results showed that the combination of acupuncture and rehabilitation was more effective than rehabilitation alone for all outcome measures. This review also suggested that acupuncture therapy was safe for the management of post-stroke shoulder pain.

Lin (2015)[3] included 13 RCTs which compared the combination of acupuncture therapies and rehabilitation to rehabilitation alone. All studies were conducted in China, with 12 of them published in Chinese and one published in English. Acupuncture therapies included body acupuncture, scalp acupuncture, abdomen acupuncture and electroacupuncture. The overall methodological quality of included RCTs was assessed as 'low' without clear criteria of judgment. Outcomes assessed by this review were pain score, FMA, activities of daily living (ADL) and adverse events (AEs). Eleven RCTs were pooled for meta-analysis, and it was found that the combination was more effective than rehabilitation for pain score (mean difference (MD): 1.50 [0.93, 2.09], I^2 = 87%), FMA (MD: 6.38 [1.16, 11.60], I^2 = 98%) and ADL (MD: 11.25 [3.00, 19.49], I^2 = 76%). Adverse events caused by acupuncture were rarely reported. This review concluded that adding acupuncture therapy to conventional rehabilitation is beneficial for the management of post-stroke shoulder pain.

Shoulder-hand Syndrome

Lu (2009)[4] included three RCTs evaluating the combination of acupuncture therapy and rehabilitation. All three studies were conducted in China and published in Chinese. Two RCTs used body acupuncture and another study evaluated electroacupuncture. Using Jadad Scores to assess the methodology quality, all three studies were assessed as 'low quality'. Outcome measures reported by these three studies were FMA (one study), ROM (one study) and effective rate (two studies). Meta-analysis could not be conducted. This review did not provide promising evidence of acupuncture therapy.

Xu (2013)[5] evaluated 21 RCTs of acupuncture therapy; 18 studies compared the combination of acupuncture and rehabilitation to rehabilitation alone, and three studies compared acupuncture to rehabilitation. All studies were conducted in China and published in Chinese. The Cochrane risk of bias assessment was used to assess the methodological quality. Overall, the included studies were of low quality. Outcomes reported by the included studies were FMA (16 studies), VAS (nine studies), ADL (six studies), ROM (one study) and effective rate (two studies). Meta-analyses showed that combining acupuncture with rehabilitation achieved better effect than rehabilitation alone for FMA, VAS and ADL. No adverse effects related to acupuncture were detected. This review concluded that adding acupuncture to conventional rehabilitation could achieve better effect for post-stroke shoulder-hand syndrome (SHS).

A recent published systematic review[6] evaluated seven RCTs; four of them compared acupuncture to rehabilitation, two compared acupuncture plus routine care to rehabilitation plus routine care, and another one compared acupuncture to CHM steaming therapy. Overall the included studies were of low quality according to the risk of bias assessment. Outcome measures included FMA (five studies), VAS (four studies), ADL (three studies) and effective rate. Meta-analysis showed that acupuncture was not significantly different to rehabilitation for FMA (MD: −0.78 [−4.58, 3.01]), ADL (MD: 3.76 [−4.94, 12.46]) and effective rate (RR: 1.11 [0.96, 1.29]); while the combination of acupuncture and rehabilitation was more effective than rehabilitation alone for VAS (MD: −2.13 [−3.63, −0.62]) and effective rate (RR: 1.27 [1.02, 1.59]). All included studies did not report information on AEs. This review did not provide conclusive evidence of acupuncture for post-stroke shoulder-hand syndrome due to the small sample size and low quality of included studies.

Identification of Clinical Studies

A total of 37,141 citations was identified after searching Chinese databases and English databases. At the end, 135 studies were included in this section, with 101 RCTs, three controlled trials and 31 non-controlled studies.

All studies were conducted in China. Over 8,000 participants were observed in these studies. Evidence from RCTs and controlled clinical trials (CCTs) was pooled to evaluate the efficacy and safety of acupuncture therapies. Results from non-controlled studies were presented descriptively.

Of the 101 RCTs, 15 studies investigated acupuncture therapies for shoulder subluxation, 24 studies focused on shoulder pain and the remaining 62 studies were of SHS. A broad range of acupuncture therapies were used; the most common were body acupuncture, electroacupuncture, acupressure, moxibustion, scalp acupuncture, floating acupuncture and some of their combinations (Fig. 7.1).

In addition, 16 studies were identified as acupuncture-related therapies not commonly practised outside of China; they will not be presented in this chapter.

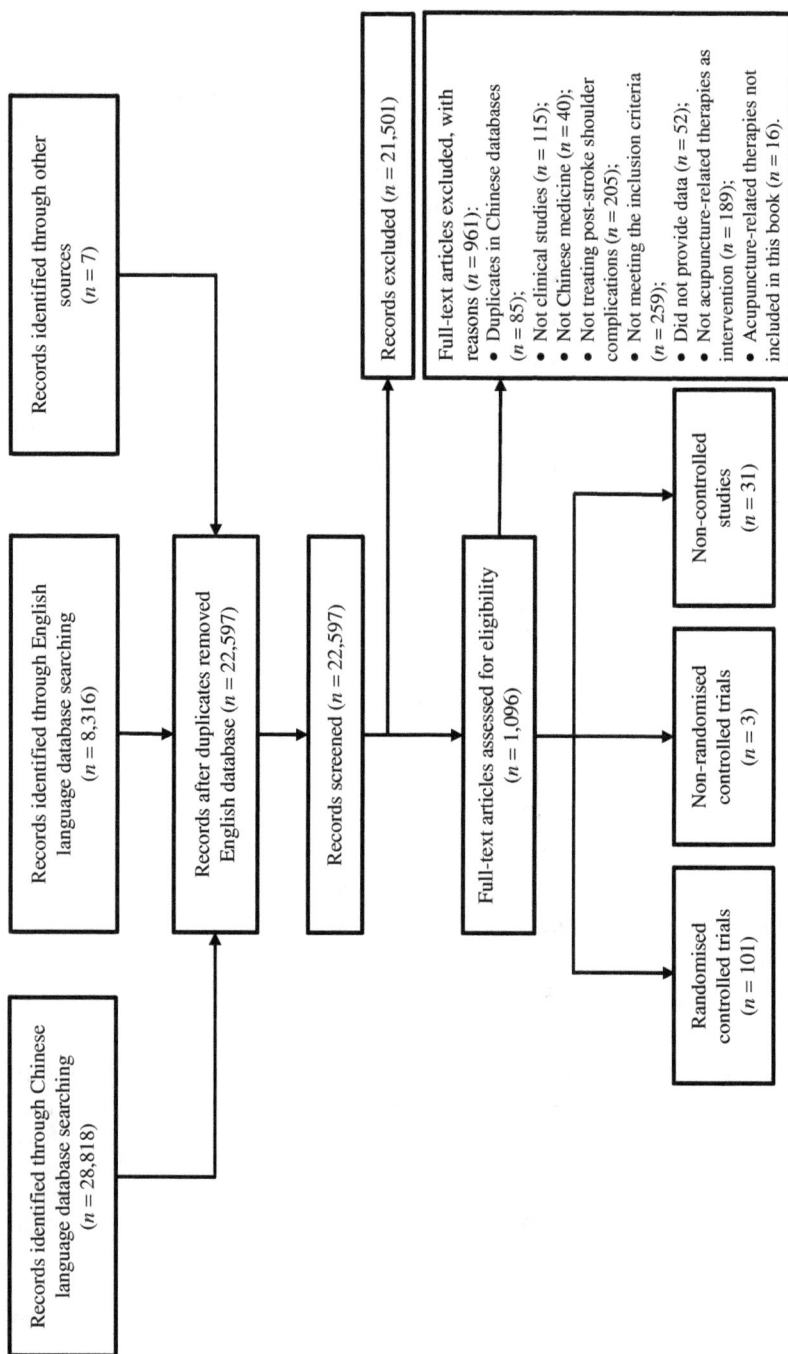

Fig. 7.1 Flowchart of study selection process: Acupuncture and related therapies.

Shoulder Subluxation

Fifteen RCTs, two CCTs and four non-controlled studies were identified.

Randomised Controlled Trials of Acupuncture

Fifteen RCTs (A1–A15), involving 930 participants, investigated acupuncture therapies for shoulder subluxation. All studies were conducted in mainland China (A1–A14) except for one study which was conducted in Taiwan (A15). These articles were published between 2000 and 2014.

All these studies were designed to evaluate the combination of acupuncture therapies with routine rehabilitation compared to routine rehabilitation alone. The treatment duration ranged from two weeks (A5) to 12 weeks (A6). Acupuncture therapies used in these studies varied, including body acupuncture (A6, A10, A13), electroacupuncture (A2–A5, A15), acupressure (A1), scalp acupuncture (A7–A9, A14) and the combination of body acupuncture and scalp acupuncture (A11, A12). The comparator was routine rehabilitation, including physical therapy, occupational therapy and Bobath exercise. Four studies only reported data of effective rate or Brunstrom scale, without mentioning our pre-defined outcomes (A5, A7–A9). The most commonly reported acupuncture points were LI15 *Jianyu* 肩髃, TE14 *Jianliao* 肩髎, SI9 *Jianzhen* 肩贞 and LI14 *Binao* 臂臑.

Risk of Bias

All these studies were described as RCTs. Only five studies reported 'using a random number table for random sequence generation' and therefore they were assessed as low risk. One study was assessed as high risk of bias due to using incorrect randomisation method. All these studies did not describe allocation concealment details, and blinding of participants and personnel (acupuncturists) was not performed. Blinding of outcome assessors was judged as unclear risk for all studies due to lack of information. The majority of studies were

Table 7.1   Risk of Bias of Randomised Controlled Trials

Risk of Bias Domain	Low Risk n (%)	Unclear Risk n (%)	High Risk n (%)
Sequence generation	5 (33.3)	9 (60)	1 (6.7)
Allocation concealment	0	15 (100)	0
Blinding of participants	0	0	15 (100)
Blinding of personnel*	0	0	15 (100)
Blinding of outcome assessors	0	15 (100)	0
Incomplete outcome data	14 (93.3)	1 (6.7)	0
Selective outcome reporting	0	15 (100)	0

*Blinding of personnel (acupuncturists) is challenging in manual therapies.

assessed as low risk for incomplete outcome data, except one study which did not provide information. All these studies were judged as unclear risk for selective outcome reporting as protocols or trial registration could not be identified for them. See Table 7.1 for details.

Outcomes

The majority of studies reported data on FMA, VAS, ADL and effective rate. It is worth noting that, being an important outcome measure for shoulder subluxation, acromiohumeral interval (AHI) was reported in two studies (A1, A13). In addition, one study reported neural dysfunction scale (NDS) (A11). The effects are presented below under each outcome measure and the meta-analyses results are summarised in Table 7.2.

Fugl-Meyer Assessment (Upper Limb)

Three studies (A6, A10, A13) reported acupuncture combined with rehabilitation therapies compared to rehabilitation alone; meta-analysis showed that there was no statistical significant difference between the combination and rehabilitation alone (MD: 5.52 [–2.56, 13.59], I^2 = 90%). Adding electroacupuncture to rehabilitation improved upper limb motor function assessed by FMA compared to rehabilitation alone in two studies (A2, A4) (MD: 8.25 [6.52, 9.97],

Table 7.2   Acupuncture as Integrative Medicine vs. Rehabilitation

Intervention	Outcome	No. of Studies	No. of Participants	Effect Size MD [95% CI]	I² %	Included Studies
Acupuncture plus rehabilitation	FMA	3	140	5.52 [–2.56, 13.59]	90	A6, A10, A13
Electroacupuncture plus rehabilitation	FMA	2	120	8.25 [6.52, 9.97]*	0	A2, A4
	Pain VAS	2	80	–1.41 [–2.16, –0.66]*	0	A3, A15

*Statistically significant. Abbreviations: CI, confidence interval; FMA, Fugl-Meyer Assessment; MD, mean difference; VAS, visual analogue scale.

I² = 0%). In one study (A12), acupuncture plus scalp acupuncture adding to rehabilitation was superior to rehabilitation alone (MD: 4.94 [0.64, 9.24]). One study (A14) that compared scalp acupuncture plus rehabilitation with rehabilitation alone also showed superior effects with regard to the combination therapy (MD: 4.19 [1.41, 6.97]). There was no statistical significant difference between acupressure plus rehabilitation and rehabilitation alone for FMA in one study (A1) (MD: 1.50 [–4.42, 7.42]).

Pain: Visual Analogue Scale

Two included studies (A3, A15) reported data on pain VAS when electroacupuncture was combined with rehabilitation. Meta-analysis showed that the combination therapy was more effective than rehabilitation alone (MD: –1.41 [–2.16, –0.66], I² = 0%).

In one study (A1), acupressure combined with rehabilitation compared to rehabilitation alone also showed a significant add-on effect (MD: –0.80 [–1.29, –0.31]).

Activities of Daily Living

Assessing the ADL by BI or Modified BI (MBI), one study (A6) showed that acupuncture combined with rehabilitation can improve 19.00 units compared with rehabilitation (MD: 19.00 [14.81, 23.19]). Also, electroacupuncture plus rehabilitation was more effective than rehabilitation alone in one study (A2) (MD: 33.20 [27.59, 38.81]).

Further, one study (A14) compared scalp acupuncture plus rehabilitation with rehabilitation alone, and the results showed that the combination achieved greater effects than rehabilitation alone (MD: 6.97 [1.30, 12.64]).

Acromiohumeral Interval

In terms of AHI, one study (A13) showed that there were no statistical significant differences between acupuncture combined with rehabilitation and rehabilitation alone (MD: −0.50 [−1.92, 0.92]). In another study (A1), acupressure combined with rehabilitation was superior to rehabilitation alone for AHI (MD: −2.50 [−4.21, −0.79]).

Neural Dysfunction Scale

One study (A11) was included in the analysis of NDS. Acupuncture plus scalp acupuncture and rehabilitation reduced NDS, compared with rehabilitation alone (MD: −3.46 [−4.81, −2.11]).

Two studies (A2, A4) combined in a meta-analysis showed a favourable effect in FMA for electroacupuncture. Commonly reported acupuncture points were LI15 *Jianyu* 肩髃, GB21 *Jianjing* 肩井, SI11 *Tianzong* 天宗 and SI9 *Jianzhen* 肩贞. Also, two studies (A3, A15) showed the favourable effect in VAS for electroacupuncture. Commonly reported acupuncture points were LI15 *Jianyu* 肩髃, GB21 *Jianjing* 肩井, TE14 *Jianliao* 肩髎 and LI14 *Binao* 臂臑.

Assessment Using GRADE

Summary of findings tables were prepared for the comparisons of acupuncture plus rehabilitation vs. rehabilitation alone, and electroacupuncture plus rehabilitation vs. rehabilitation alone. The evidence of benefit of adding acupuncture to rehabilitation for ADL, and the evidence of positive add-on effects of electroacupuncture for FMA, VAS and ADL were all assessed as 'low' certainty. See Tables 7.3 and 7.4 for details.

Table 7.3 GRADE: Acupuncture Plus Routine Rehabilitation vs. Routine Rehabilitation for Post-stroke Shoulder Subluxation

Outcomes	No. of Participants (Studies) Follow-up	Certainty of the Evidence (GRADE)	Risk with Rehabilitation	Risk Difference with Acupuncture + Rehabilitation
			Anticipated Absolute Effects	
FMA	140 (3 RCTs)	⊕◯◯◯ VERY LOW[a,b,c]	The mean FMA was **28.09** points	MD **5.52 points higher** (2.56 lower to 13.59 higher)
ADL	60 (1 RCT)	⊕⊕◯◯ LOW[a,d]	The mean ADL was **63.83** points	MD **19 points higher** (14.81 higher to 23.19 higher)
AHI	40 (1 RCT)	⊕◯◯◯ VERY LOW[a,c]	The mean AHI was **12.59** mm	MD **0.5 mm lower** (1.92 lower to 0.92 higher)

The risk in the intervention group (and its 95% confidence interval) is based on the assumed risk in the comparison group and the relative effect of the intervention (and its 95% CI).

Abbreviations: ADL, activities of daily living; AHI, acromiohumeral interval; CI, confidence interval; FMA, Fugl-Meyer Assessment; GRADE, Grading of Recommendations Assessment, Development and Evaluation; MD, mean difference; RCT, randomised control trial; VAS, visual analogue scale.

Notes:

a. Lack of blinding of participants and personnel.
b. Considerable statistical heterogeneity.
c. Small sample size limits certainty of results and 95% CI overlaps no effect.
d. Small sample size limits certainty of results.

Study References:

FMA: A6, A10, A13
ADL: A6
AHI: A13

Table 7.4 GRADE: Electroacupuncture Plus Routine Rehabilitation vs. Routine Rehabilitation for Post-stroke Shoulder Subluxation

Outcomes	No. of Participants (Studies) Follow-up	Certainty of the Evidence (GRADE)	Risk with Rehabilitation	Anticipated Absolute Effects
				Risk Difference with Electroacupuncture + Rehabilitation
FMA	120 (2 RCTs)	⊕⊕◯◯ LOW[a,b]	The mean FMA was **18.55** points	MD **8.25 points higher** (6.52 higher to 9.97 higher)
Pain VAS	80 (2 RCTs)	⊕⊕◯◯ LOW[a,b]	The mean VAS was **3.42** points	MD **1.41 points lower** (2.16 lower to 0.66 lower)
ADL	60 (1 RCT)	⊕⊕◯◯ LOW[a,b]	The mean ADL was **43.3** points	MD **33.2 points higher** (27.59 higher to 38.81 higher)

The risk in the intervention group (and its 95% confidence interval) is based on the assumed risk in the comparison group and the relative effect of the intervention (and its 95% CI).

Abbreviations: ADL, activities of daily living; CI, confidence interval; FMA, Fugl-Meyer Assessment; GRADE, Grading of Recommendations Assessment, Development and Evaluation; MD, mean difference; RCT, randomised control trial; VAS, visual analogue scale.

Notes:

a. Lack of blinding of participants and personnel.
b. Small sample size limits certainty of results.

Study References:

FMA: A2, A4
Pain VAS: A3, A15
ADL: A2

Controlled Clinical Trials (Non-randomised) of Acupuncture

Two non-randomised controlled studies (A16, A17), including 122 participants, evaluated acupuncture therapies. One study (A17) evaluated electroacupuncture combined with rehabilitation compared to rehabilitation alone; the results showed that adding electroacupuncture could improve upper limb function assessed using FMA (MD: 10.84 [5.37, 16.31]) and ADL (MD: 10.29 [5.50, 15.08]). In addition, effective rate and Brunnstrom scale were reported in another study (A16), which compared acupuncture plus rehabilitation with rehabilitation alone. These data were not further analysed.

Non-controlled Studies of Acupuncture

Four non-controlled studies, including 225 participants, evaluated the acupuncture therapies for shoulder subluxation (A18–A21). All studies were case series evaluating the combination of electroacupuncture and rehabilitation. Fifteen different acupuncture points were used in these studies and the most common ones were LI15 *Jianyu* 肩髃, TE14 *Jianliao* 肩髎, LI14 *Binao* 臂臑, GB21 *Jianjing* 肩井, SI11 *Tianzong* 天宗 and SI13 *Quyuan* 曲垣.

Safety of Acupuncture Therapies for Shoulder Subluxation

Information on AEs was mentioned by one study (A12), reporting that there was no AE occurring. Acupuncture-related therapies appear to be well tolerated by people with shoulder subluxation.

Shoulder Pain

Acupuncture therapies for post-stroke shoulder pain were evaluated in 24 RCTs published by 25 articles (A22–A46: A24 and A25 are from the same study), one non-randomised CCT (A47) and six non-controlled studies (A48–A53).

Randomised Controlled Trials of Acupuncture

Twenty-four RCTs, involving 1,512 participants, evaluated the effects of acupuncture therapies for post-stroke shoulder pain. All studies were conducted in China and published between 2006 and 2014.

Of these studies, one study (A40) compared acupuncture to rehabilitation, one study (A43) evaluated scalp acupuncture and body acupuncture compared with topical medication (Diclofenac); the other 22 studies (A22–A39, A41, A42, A44–A46) evaluated the add-on effects of acupuncture therapies to routine rehabilitation. The treatment duration ranged from ten days (A33) to 60 days (A28). Acupuncture therapies used in these 24 RCTs varied, including body acupuncture (nine studies) (A30, A31, A37–A40, A42, A45, A46), electroacupuncture (four studies including five articles) (A24–A27, A41), acupuncture plus moxibustion (two studies) (A35, A36), moxibustion (two studies) (A22, A23), body acupuncture plus scalp acupuncture (three studies) (A32, A43, A44), floating acupuncture 浮针 (two studies) (A28, A29) and wrist-ankle acupuncture 腕踝针 (two studies) (A33, A34). The latter two therapies were developed recently and are not commonly used in clinical practice. Used as comparators, rehabilitation therapy included physical therapy, occupational therapy, Bobath exercise, and their combinations. The majority of studies reported one of our pre-defined outcomes, including FMA, VAS or ADL. Five studies only reported effective rate to assess the effect of acupuncture-related therapies (A29, A32, A34, A41, A43).

The duration of treatment ranged from ten days (A33) to three months (A42). The most commonly reported acupuncture points were LI15 *Jianyu* 肩髃, TE14 *Jianliao* 肩髎 and SI9 *Jianzhen* 肩贞.

Risk of Bias

All studies were described as RCTs, ten studies reported an appropriate method for sequence generation and were assessed as 'low' risk of bias, and others were 'unclear' risk. Only one study (A30) was judged as 'low' risk for allocation concealment, since it used sealed

Table 7.5   Risk of Bias of Randomised Controlled Trials

Risk of Bias Domain	Low Risk *n* (%)	Unclear Risk *n* (%)	High Risk *n* (%)
Sequence generation	10 (41.7)	14 (58.3)	0 (100)
Allocation concealment	1 (4.2)	23 (95.8)	0 (100)
Blinding of participants	0 (100)	0 (100)	24 (100)
Blinding of personnel	0 (100)	0 (100)	24 (100)
Blinding of outcome assessors	0 (100)	24 (100)	0 (100)
Incomplete outcome data	19 (79.1)	4 (16.7)	1 (4.2)
Selective outcome reporting	0 (100)	24 (100)	0 (100)

Note: Blinding of personnel (acupuncturists) is challenging in manual therapies.

envelopes to conceal group allocation. None of the studies made an effort to blind participants and personnel (acupuncturists). Blinding of outcome assessors was judged as 'unclear' risk for all studies due to lack of information. One study (A38) was rated as 'high' risk of bias for incomplete outcome data due to high drop-out rate, four studies were judged as 'unclear' risk because of lack of information. Selective outcome reporting was judged as 'unclear' risk for all studies as none of the trials was registered or had published their protocols. See Table 7.5 for details.

Outcomes

The outcomes of FMA (upper limb), pain VAS and ADL were commonly used in the majority of studies. Two studies (A25, A27) evaluated pain with a numerical rating scale (NRS). One study reported NDS (A44). The effects of acupuncture therapies are presented below under each outcome, and the meta-analyses results are summarised in Table 7.6.

Fugl-Meyer Assessment (Upper Limb)

Fugl-Meyer Assessment was used to measure the upper limb motor function in 15 studies. Acupuncture combined with rehabilitation

Table 7.6   Acupuncture as Integrative Medicine vs. Rehabilitation

Intervention	Outcome	No. of Studies	No. of Participants	Effect Size MD [95% CI]	I²	Included Studies
Acupuncture plus rehabilitation	FMA	6	332	6.34 [4.47, 8.20]*	0	A30, A37–A39, A45, A46
	Pain VAS	7	432	–2.14 [–2.50, –1.77]*	40	A30, A37–A39, A42, A45, A46
	ADL	4	182	17.30 [12.67, 21.93]*	0	A30, A38, A39, A45
Electroacupuncture plus rehabilitation	FMA	2	168	12.89 [4.23, 21.54]*	88	A24, A25, A27
	Pain NRS	2	168	–2.15 [–4.05, –0.25]*	94	A25, A27
Acupuncture plus moxibustion and rehabilitation	FMA	2	84	8.38[–15.41, 32.16]	100	A35, A36
	Pain VAS	2	84	–2.17 [–3.34, –0.99]*	84	A35, A36
Moxibustion plus rehabilitation	Pain VAS	2	94	–2.44 [–3.18, –1.70]*	19	A22, A23

*Statistically significant. Abbreviations: ADL, activities of daily living; CI, confidence interval; FMA, Fugl-Meyer Assessment; MD, mean difference; NRS, numerical rating scale; VAS, visual analogue scale.

improved FMA compared with rehabilitation alone in six studies (A30, A37–A39, A45, A46) (MD: 6.34 [4.47, 8.20], I² = 0%). Two studies, reported in three articles (A24, A25, A27), investigated the effects of the combination of electroacupuncture and rehabilitation compared to rehabilitation alone. The meta-analysis showed that electroacupuncture plus rehabilitation was more effective than rehabilitation alone (MD: 12.89 [4.23, 21.54], I² = 88%). Acupuncture plus moxibustion combined with rehabilitation was not superior to rehabilitation alone, in terms of motor function measured with FMA in two studies (A35, A36) (MD: 8.38 [–15.41, 32.16], I² = 100%).

Results of single studies showed that: (1) there was no statistical significant difference between wrist-ankle acupuncture 腕踝针 plus rehabilitation and rehabilitation alone in one study (A33) (MD: 6.48 [–1.92, 14.88]); (2) the combination of moxibustion and rehabilitation showed additional benefit compared to rehabilitation alone

(A22) (MD: 15.40 [7.20, 23.60]); (3) floating acupuncture 浮针 was superior to rehabilitation when combined with the same rehabilitation (A28) (MD: 10.22 [4.22, 16.22]) and (4) acupuncture alone was superior for upper limb motor function compared to rehabilitation (A40) (MD: 4.50 [2.81, 6.19]).

Pain: Visual Analogue Scale

When acupuncture was combined with rehabilitation, the meta-analysis showed significantly superior effects in pain relief compared to rehabilitation alone in seven studies (A30, A37–A39, A42, A45, A46) (MD: –2.14 [–2.50, –1.77], $I^2 = 40\%$). Two studies (A35, A36) reported pain VAS with acupuncture plus moxibustion combined with rehabilitation; meta-analysis showed benefits compared to rehabilitation alone (MD: –2.17 [–3.34, –0.99], $I^2 = 84\%$). Pain VAS was reduced by combining moxibustion with rehabilitation, compared to rehabilitation alone, in two studies (A22, A23) (MD: –2.44 [–3.18, –1.70], $I^2 = 19\%$).

In addition, there are also some single studies which showed that: (1) electroacupuncture combined with rehabilitation was superior to rehabilitation for pain VAS (A26) (MD: –1.26 [–2.07, –0.45]); (2) acupuncture alone showed a mild superior effect in reducing pain compared to rehabilitation (A40) (MD: –1.23 [–1.92, –0.54]) and (3) in one study that evaluated the effect of floating acupuncture combined with rehabilitation, the pain VAS was significantly lower in the combination therapy compared to rehabilitation alone (A28) (MD: –3.19 [–3.75, –2.63]).

Pain: Numerical Rating Scale

Two studies (A25, A27) measured pain using NRS. The results showed electroacupuncture combined with rehabilitation was superior to rehabilitation alone (MD: –2.15 [–4.05, –0.25], $I^2 = 94\%$).

Activities of Daily Living

Activities of daily living were evaluated using BI in three studies (A23, A25, A33) and MBI in four studies (A30, A38, A39, A45). Four studies (A30, A38, A39, A45) showed that acupuncture combined with rehabilitation improved MBI compared with rehabilitation alone (MD: 17.30 [12.67, 21.93], I^2 = 0%). Electroacupuncture compared with rehabilitation improved 9.62 units in one study (A25) when combined with rehabilitation (MD: 9.62 [0.70, 18.54]).

Barthel Index was improved significantly at the end of treatment with moxibustion plus rehabilitation, compared with rehabilitation alone, in one study (A23) (MD: 14.11 [10.63, 17.59]). Also, wrist-ankle acupuncture 腕踝针 combined with rehabilitation improved BI compared with rehabilitation alone in one study (A33) (MD: 8.22 [0.24, 16.20]).

Neural Dysfunction Scale

In one study (A44), the combination of acupuncture plus scalp acupuncture and rehabilitation was superior to rehabilitation alone (MD: −4.41 [−5.40, −3.42]).

The most frequent acupuncture points used in studies from favourable meta-analyses were calculated (see Table 7.7). Studies were grouped according to the outcome measures (FMA, ADL or pain VAS/NRS), and regardless of their comparator (rehabilitation therapy alone or with pharmacotherapy).

Assessment Using GRADE

A summary of findings table was prepared for the comparison of acupuncture plus rehabilitation vs. rehabilitation alone (Table 7.8). Adding acupuncture to rehabilitation could improve treatment effects for FMA and pain VAS, with evidence of 'moderate' quality. Acupuncture also showed add-on effects to rehabilitation for ADL; however, this evidence is of 'low' certainty.

Controlled Clinical Trials (Non-randomised) of Acupuncture

Only one non-randomised CCT evaluated acupuncture therapy (A47). It investigated the combination of acupuncture and rehabilitation in 79 participants, and reported data on the change of FMA and pain VAS.

Table 7.7 Frequently Reported Acupuncture Points in Meta-analyses Showing Favourable Effect: Manual Acupuncture, Electroacupuncture and Acupressure

Outcome Category	No. of Meta-analyses	No. of Studies in Meta-analyses	Acupuncture Points (No. of Studies)
FMA	2	8 A24, A27, A30, A37–A39, A45, A46	TE14 Jianliao 肩髎 (4) SI9 Jianzhen 肩贞 (4) LI15 Jianyu 肩髃 (3) LI11 Quchi 曲池 (3) LI10 Shousanli 手三里 (3) TE5 Waiguan 外关 (3) CV12 Zhongwan 中脘 (3) KI17 Shangqu 商曲 (3)
Pain VAS/ NRS	3	11 A25, A27, A30, A35–A39, A42, A45, A46	TE14 Jianliao 肩髎 (5) SI9 Jianzhen 肩贞 (5) LI11 Quchi 曲池 (5) LI15 Jianyu 肩髃 (4) LI10 Shousanli 手三里 (4) TE5 Waiguan 外关 (4)
ADL	1	4 A30, A38, A39, A45	SI9 Jianzhen 肩贞 (2) SI11 Tianzong 天宗 (2) CV12 Zhongwan 中脘 (2) KI17 Shangqu 商曲 (2)

Abbreviations: ADL, activities of daily living; FMA, Fugl-Meyer Assessment; NRS, numerical rating scale; VAS, visual analogue scale.

The results showed that acupuncture combined with rehabilitation achieved greater changes compared to rehabilitation alone on FMA (MD: 1.90 [0.85, 2.95]) and Pain VAS (MD: 1.40 [0.63, 2.17]).

Non-controlled Studies of Acupuncture

Acupuncture therapies were also evaluated in six non-controlled studies. A total of 361 participants was researched in these five traditional acupuncture studies (A48–A52) and one wrist-ankle acupuncture 腕踝针 study (A53). Chinese syndrome was not reported in these studies. Over 20 different acupoints were used in these studies and the most common ones were LI15 *Jianyu* 肩髃, TE14 *Jianliao* 肩髎, SI9 *Jianzhen* 肩贞 and SI11 *Tianzong* 天宗.

Table 7.8   GRADE: Acupuncture Plus Rehabilitation Compared to Rehabilitation for Shoulder Pain

Outcomes	No. of Participants (Studies) Follow-up	Certainty of the Evidence (GRADE)	Anticipated Absolute Effects	
			Risk with Rehabilitation	Risk Difference with Acupuncture + Rehabilitation
FMA	332 (6 RCTs)	⊕⊕⊕◯ MODERATE[a]	The mean FMA was **24.42** points	MD **6.34 points higher** (4.47 higher to 8.2 higher)
Pain VAS	432 (7 RCTs)	⊕⊕⊕◯ MODERATE[a]	The mean VAS was **4.49** points	MD **2.14 points lower** (2.5 lower to 1.77 lower)
ADL	182 (4 RCTs)	⊕⊕◯◯ LOW[a,b]	The mean ADL was **51.76** points	MD **17.3 points higher** (12.67 higher to 21.93 higher)
Adverse events	100 (2 RCTs)		Two studies reported no adverse events observed.	

The risk in the intervention group (and its 95% confidence interval) is based on the assumed risk in the comparison group and the relative effect of the intervention (and its 95% CI).

Abbreviations: ADL, activities of daily living; CI, confidence interval; FMA, Fugl-Meyer Assessment; GRADE, Grading of Recommendations Assessment, Development and Evaluation; MD, mean difference; RCT, randomised control trial; VAS, visual analogue scale.

Notes:

a. Lack of blinding of participants and personnel.
b. Small sample size limits certainty of results.

Study Reference:

FMA: A30, A37–A39, A45, A46
Pain VAS: A30, A37–A39, A42, A45, A46
ADL: A30, A38, A39, A45
Adverse events: A45, A46

Safety of Acupuncture Therapies for Shoulder Pain

Five of the 24 studies (A24, A35, A41, A45, A46) reported the safety of acupuncture therapies in RCTs. Four of them (A35, A41, A45, A46) stated that no events occurred.

Only one study (A24) mentioned that several cases of subcutaneous haemorrhage occurred after electroacupuncture therapy; the mild symptom disappeared in two weeks without any additional treatment.

The non-randomised controlled study and non-controlled clinical studies did not provide any information of adverse events.

Shoulder-hand Syndrome

Acupuncture therapies for the treatment of SHS were assessed in 62 RCTs (A54–A115) and 21 non-controlled clinical studies (A116–A136).

Randomised Controlled Trials of Acupuncture

A total of 62 RCTs (A54–A115), involving 4,823 participants, investigated acupuncture therapies for SHS. All studies were conducted in China and published between 2006 and 2015.

The treatment duration ranged between ten days (A66) and eight weeks (A58) and no study reported Chinese medicine syndrome. With the exception of two RCTs (A68, A111), 60 studies investigated the add-on effects of acupuncture therapies when they were integrated with routine care and rehabilitation. These 62 studies evaluated multiple acupuncture therapies, including acupuncture (29 studies) (A54, A67–A69, A72, A74, A75, A77–A80, A83, A88–A97, A99, A101–A103, A106, A108, A115), electroacupuncture (15 studies) (A55–A60, A70, A71, A104, A105, A107, A111–A114), floating acupuncture (four studies) (A61–A64), moxibustion (two studies) (A65, A73), acupuncture and moxibustion (five studies) (A81, A85–A87, A100), scalp acupuncture and body acupuncture (five studies) (A76, A82, A98, A109, A110), wrist-ankle acupuncture 腕踝针 (one study) (A84) and acupuncture points infrared radiation (one study) (A66). Routine rehabilitation therapies were used as control methods, including physical therapy, occupational therapy, Bobath exercise, and their combinations.

In total, over 80 different points were used, with the most common ones being LI15 *Jianyu* 肩髃, LI11 *Quchi* 曲池, LI4 *Hegu* 合谷, TE5 *Waiguan* 外关, TE14 *Jianliao* 肩髎 and SI9 *Jianzhen* 肩贞.

Risk of Bias

Included studies were all described as randomised but only 18 studies introduced correct methods for sequence generation; others were of 'unclear' risk for this item. Two studies used sealed envelopes for allocation concealment; therefore they were judged as 'low' risk of bias, and the remaining studies did not describe such details. Blinding of participants and personnel (acupuncturists) was not performed in any study. Blinding of outcome assessors was judged as 'unclear' risk for all studies due to lack of information. One study described high drop out and no further analysis, so it was assessed as 'high' risk for incomplete outcome data. Two studies were 'unclear' risk due to lack of information. The majority of studies were judged as 'unclear' risk for selective outcome reporting as their protocols were not published. One study was at 'high' risk because its pre-specified outcome was not reported. See Table 7.9 for a summary.

Outcomes

The commonly reported outcomes for these 62 studies were FMA score, pain VAS, ADL and NDS. The treatment effects are presented below under each outcome measure. Results of the meta-analyses are summarised in Table 7.10.

Fugl-Meyer Assessment (Upper Limb)

Fifteen studies (A67, A72, A74, A77, A79, A80, A89, A91–A94, A97, A101, A103, A108) reported data on upper limb FMA score when acupuncture was combined with rehabilitation. Meta-analysis

Table 7.9   Risk of Bias of Randomised Controlled Trials

Risk of Bias Domain	Low Risk n (%)	Unclear Risk n (%)	High Risk n (%)
Sequence generation	18 (29)	44 (71.0)	0
Allocation concealment	2 (3.2)	60 (96.8)	0
Blinding of participants	0	0	62 (100)
Blinding of personnel	0	0	62 (100)
Blinding of outcome assessors	0	62 (100)	0
Incomplete outcome data	59 (95.2)	2 (3.2)	1 (1.6)
Selective outcome reporting	0	61 (98.4)	1 (1.6)

Note: Blinding of personnel (acupuncturists) is challenging in manual therapies.

showed that the combination of acupuncture and rehabilitation improved FMA scores compared with rehabilitation alone (MD: 7.84 [5.95, 9.72], $I^2 = 80\%$). Electroacupuncture combined with rehabilitation also showed benefits for FMA score, compared with rehabilitation in eight studies (A59, A70, A71, A105, A107, A112–A114) (MD: 10.64 [9.05, 12.23], $I^2 = 16\%$). In five studies (A76, A82, A98, A109, A110) acupuncture, plus scalp acupuncture with rehabilitation, was superior to rehabilitation alone for FMA score (MD: 7.18 [2.49, 11.86], $I^2 = 94\%$). Results from five studies (A81, A85–A87, A100) found adding acupuncture plus moxibustion to rehabilitation improved 12.57 units in FMA score (MD: 12.57 [10.45, 14.68], $I^2 = 94\%$).

In addition, moxibustion was superior to rehabilitation in one study (A65) (MD: 2.33 [0.55, 4.11]). Significant add-on effects to rehabilitation were also seen in meta-analysis of two studies (A63, A64) for floating acupuncture (MD: 8.14 [4.92, 11.35], $I^2 = 38\%$), and one study (A84) for wrist-ankle acupuncture (MD: 8.51 [6.05, 10.97]) (Table 7.10).

Pain Visual Analogue Scale

Acupuncture combined with rehabilitation reduced pain score compared to rehabilitation alone in 12 studies (A67, A72, A74, A80, A83,

Table 7.10   Acupuncture as Integrative Medicine vs. Rehabilitation

Intervention	Outcome	No. of Studies	No. of Participants	Effect Size MD [95% CI]	I² (%)	Included Studies
Acupuncture plus rehabilitation	FMA	15	1410	7.84 [5.95, 9.72]*	80	A67, A72, A74, A77, A79, A80, A89, A91–A94, A97, A101, A103, A108
	Pain VAS	12	1059	−1.73 [−2.19, −1.27]*	91	A67, A72, A74, A80, A83, A88, A89, A93, A94, A102, A106, A108
	ADL	7	567	10.32 [4.46, 16.17]*	88	A79, A93, A96, A102, A103, A106, A108
	NDS	3	240	−4.43 [−5.01, −3.85]*	0	A92, A98, A110
Electroacupuncture plus rehabilitation	FMA	8	523	10.64 [9.05, 12.23]*	16	A59, A70, A71, A105, A107, A112–A114
	Pain VAS	9	509	−1.55 [−1.91, −1.19]*	55	A55, A57, A70, A71, A105, A107, A112–A114
	ADL	5	304	8.27 [3.88, 12.65]*	70	A57, A59, A104, A107, A113
Acupuncture plus scalp acupuncture plus rehabilitation	FMA	5	318	7.18 [2.49, 11.86]*	94	A76, A82, A98, A109, A110
	Pain VAS	3	180	−1.09 [−1.56, −0.62]*	28	A98, A109, A110
Acupuncture plus moxibustion plus rehabilitation	FMA	5	386	12.57 [10.45, 14.68]*	94	A81, A85–A87, A100
	Pain VAS	4	306	−1.55 [−1.78, −1.32]*	38	A81, A85–A87
	ADL	2	180	15.81 [10.47, 21.15]*	79	A81, A86
Floating acupuncture plus rehabilitation	FMA	2	140	8.14 [4.92, 11.35]*	38	A63, A64
	Pain VAS	4	240	−1.86 [−2.52, −1.19]*	82	A61–A64

*Statistically significant. Abbreviations: ADL, activities of daily living; CI, confidence interval; FMA, Fugl-Meyer Assessment; MD, mean difference; NDS, neural dysfunction scale; VAS, visual analogue scale.

A88, A89, A93, A94, A102, A106, A108) (MD: −1.73 [−2.19, −1.27], I² = 91%). Nine studies (A55, A57. A70, A71, A105, A107, A112–A114) assessed pain VAS for comparing electroacupuncture plus rehabilitation to rehabilitation alone; the results from the meta-analysis favoured the combination therapy (MD: −1.55 [−1.91, −1.19], I^2 = 55%). When body acupuncture plus scalp acupuncture were combined with rehabilitation in three studies (A98, A109, A110), pain VAS score was significantly lower than that of rehabilitation alone (MD: −1.09 [−1.56, −0.62], I^2 = 28%). Four studies (A81, A85, A86, A87), involving 306 participants, evaluated pain VAS for acupuncture combined with moxibustion and rehabilitation; the meta-analysis showed significant benefit of the combination of acupuncture, moxibustion and rehabilitation compared to rehabilitation alone (MD: −1.55 [−1.78, −1.32], I^2 = 38%).

One single study showed that moxibustion was more effective than rehabilitation for pain score (MD: −1.51 [−2.22, −0.80]). Floating acupuncture was shown to have add-on effect for pain VAS by meta-analysis of four studies (A61–A64) (MD: −1.86 [−2.52, −1.19], I^2 = 82%), as well as wrist-ankle acupuncture by one study (A84) (MD: −1.43 [−2.20, −0.66]) (Table 7.10).

Activities of Daily Living

Most of the studies evaluated ADL using BI or MBI as outcome measures. Seventeen studies (A57, A59, A61, A68, A79, A81, A86, A93, A96, A102–A104, A106–A109, A113) reported data on ADL. Acupuncture combined with rehabilitation improved ADL in seven studies (A79, A93, A96, A102, A103, A106, A108) (MD: 10.32 [4.46, 16.17], I^2 = 88%). When electroacupuncture plus rehabilitation was compared with rehabilitation alone in five studies (A57, A59, A104, A107, A113), the combination showed superior effects compared to rehabilitation alone (MD: 8.27 [3.88, 12.65], I^2 = 70%). Meta-analysis of two studies (A86, A81) also showed that acupuncture combined with moxibustion plus rehabilitation was superior to rehabilitation alone for ADL (MD: 15.81 [10.47, 21.15], I^2 = 79%).

One study (A109) showed benefit in BI when adding acupuncture plus scalp acupuncture to rehabilitation (MD: 9.33 [1.14, 17.52]). One study (A68) compared acupuncture alone to rehabilitation; there was no statistically significant difference between acupuncture and rehabilitation for ADL (MD: 6.96 [−2.58, 16.50]). The effect of floating acupuncture was assessed in one study comparing with western medicine (A61). This study showed that acupuncture was more effective than medication (MD: 8.97 [3.70, 14.24]).

Neural Dysfunction Scale

Three studies (A92, A98, A110) reported on NDS. Meta-analysis showed that the combination of acupuncture and rehabilitation was more effective than rehabilitation alone (MD: −4.43 [−5.01, −3.85], $I^2 = 0\%$).

The most frequent acupuncture points used in those studies included in favourable meta-analyses were calculated (Table 7.11). Studies were grouped according to the outcome measures and regardless of their comparator (rehabilitation therapy alone or with pharmacotherapy).

Assessment Using GRADE

Summary of findings tables were prepared for the comparisons of acupuncture plus rehabilitation vs. rehabilitation alone, and electroacupuncture plus rehabilitation vs. rehabilitation alone. The evidence of benefit of adding acupuncture to rehabilitation for FMA, pain VAS and ADL was assessed as 'low' certainty, while the evidence of positive add-on effects of electroacupuncture for the three outcomes were of 'moderate' or 'low' certainty. See Tables 7.12 and 7.13 for details.

Non-controlled Studies of Acupuncture

Twenty-one non-controlled studies (A116–A136), involving 801 participants, were identified evaluating acupuncture therapy for post-stroke SHS. All these studies were conducted in China, which included 20 case series (A116–A132, A134–A136) and one case report (A133). Acupuncture therapies evaluated by these studies include body acupuncture (eight studies, A116, A124, A125, A127, A132, A134–A136), electroacupuncture (five studies, A118–A120,

Table 7.11   Frequently Reported Acupuncture Points in Meta-analyses Showing Favourable Effect: Manual Acupuncture, Electroacupuncture and Acupressure

Outcome Category	No. of Meta-analyses	No. of Studies in Meta-analyses	Acupuncture Points (No. of Studies)
FMA	3	29 A59, A67, A70–A72, A74, A77, A79–A81, A85–A89, A91–A94, A97, A100, A101, A103, A105, A107, A108, A112–A114	LI11 Quchi 曲池 (16) LI4 Hegu 合谷 (15) TE5 Waiguan 外关 (15) LI15 Jianyu 肩髃 (14) LI10 Shousanli 手三里 (11) PC6 Neiguan 内关 (10) TE14 Jianliao 肩髎 (7) HT1 Jiquan 极泉 (6) SI9 Jianzhen 肩贞 (5) LU5 Chize 尺泽 (5)
Pain VAS	3	25 A55, A57, A67, A70–A72, A74, A80, A81, A83, A85–A89, A93, A94, A102, A105–A108, A112–A114	LI15 Jianyu 肩髃 (13) LI4 Hegu 合谷 (12) TE5 Waiguan 外关 (12) LI11 Quchi 曲池 (11) LI10 Shousanli 手三里 (9) PC6 Neiguan 内关 (8) TE14 Jianliao 肩髎 (6) SI9 Jianzhen 肩贞 (5)
ADL	3	14 A57, A59, A79, A81, A86, A93, A96, A102–A104, A106–A108, A113	LI15 Jianyu 肩髃 (12) TE5 Waiguan 外关 (10) LI10 Shousanli 手三里 (9) LI4 Hegu 合谷 (9) PC6 Neiguan 内关 (9) LI11 Quchi 曲池 (8) TE14 Jianliao 肩髎 (6)
NDS	1	3 A92, A98, A110	LI15 Jianyu 肩髃 (2) LI11 Quchi 曲池 (2) TE5 Waiguan 外关 (2)

Abbreviations: ADL, activities of daily living; FMA, Fugl-Meyer Assessment; NDS, neural dysfunction scale; VAS, visual analogue scale.

A130, A131), acupuncture plus moxibustion (two studies, A117, A126), moxibustion (two studies, A123, A133) and one study each for acupuncture plus fomentation (A129), floating acupuncture (A122), scalp acupuncture plus body acupuncture (A128) and

Table 7.12 GRADE: Acupuncture Plus Rehabilitation Compared to Rehabilitation for Shoulder-hand Syndrome

Outcomes	No. of Participants (Studies) Follow-up	Certainty of the Evidence (GRADE)	Anticipated Absolute Effects	
			Risk with Rehabilitation	Risk Difference with Acupuncture + Rehabilitation
FMA	1410 (15 RCTs)	⊕⊕◯◯ LOW[a,b]	The mean FMA was **36.19** points	MD **7.84 points higher** (5.95 higher to 9.72 higher)
Pain VAS	1059 (12 RCTs)	⊕⊕◯◯ LOW[a,b]	The mean VAS was **4.29** points	MD **1.73 points lower** (2.19 lower to 1.27 lower)
ADL	567 (7 RCTs)	⊕⊕◯◯ LOW[a,b]	The mean ADL was **48.94** points	MD **10.32 points higher** (4.46 higher to 16.17 higher)
Adverse events	82 (1 RCT)		One study reported no adverse events observed.	

The risk in the intervention group (and its 95% confidence interval) is based on the assumed risk in the comparison group and the relative effect of the intervention (and its 95% CI).

Abbreviations: ADL, activities of daily living; CI, confidence interval; FMA, Fugl-Meyer Assessment; GRADE, Grading of Recommendations Assessment, Development and Evaluation; MD, mean difference; RCT, randomised control trial; VAS, visual analogue scale.

Notes:

a. Lack of blinding of participants and personnel.
b. Considerable statistical heterogeneity.

Study Reference:

FMA: A67, A72, A74, A77, A79, A80, A89, A91–A94, A97, A101, A103, A108
Pain VAS: A67, A72, A74, A80, A83, A88, A89, A93, A94, A102, A106, A108
ADL: A79, A93, A96, A102, A103, A106, A108
Adverse events: A67

Table 7.13 GRADE: Electroacupuncture Plus Rehabilitation Compared to Rehabilitation for Shoulder-hand Syndrome

Outcomes	No. of Participants (Studies) Follow-up	Certainty of the Evidence (GRADE)	Anticipated Absolute Effects	
			Risk with Rehabilitation	Risk Difference with Electroacupuncture + Rehabilitation
FMA	523 (8 RCTs)	⊕⊕⊕◯ MODERATE[a,b]	The mean FMA was 32.26 points	MD **10.64 points higher** (9.05 higher to 12.23 higher)
Pain VAS	509 (9 RCTs)	⊕⊕◯◯ LOW[a,b]	The mean VAS was 3.79 points	MD **1.55 points lower** (1.91 lower to 1.19 lower)
ADL	304 (5 RCTs)	⊕⊕◯◯ LOW[a,b]	The mean ADL was 58.00 points	MD **8.27 points higher** (3.88 higher to 12.65 higher)
Adverse events	132 (2 RCTs)		One study reported no adverse events observed; another study reported that three cases and two cases experienced subcutaneous haemorrhage in the electroacupuncture group and rehabilitation group respectively. The events were mild and solved after external application.	

The risk in the intervention group (and its 95% confidence interval) is based on the assumed risk in the comparison group and the relative effect of the intervention (and its 95% CI).

Abbreviations: ADL, activities of daily living; CI, confidence interval; FMA, Fugl-Meyer Assessment; GRADE, Grading of Recommendations Assessment, Development and Evaluation; MD, mean difference; RCT, randomised control trial; VAS, visual analogue scale.

Notes:

a. Lack of blinding of participants and personnel.
b. Moderate statistical heterogeneity.

Study Reference:

FMA: A59, A70, A71, A105, A107, A112–A114
Pain VAS: A55, A57, A70, A71, A105, A107, A112–A114
ADL: A57, A59, A104, A107, A113
Adverse events: A112, A114

acupuncture plus electrostimulation (A121). None of these studies reported the Chinese syndrome for this post-stroke complication. Over 40 different acupuncture points were used in the studies, with the most common ones being LI15 *Jianyu* 肩髃, LI11 *Quchi* 曲池, LI10 *Shousanli* 手三里, TE5 *Waiguan* 外关, LI4 *Hegu* 合谷, PC6 *Neiguan* 内关, LI14 *Binao* 臂臑, TE14 *Jianliao* 肩髎, SI9 *Jianzhen* 肩贞 and HT1 *Jiquan* 极泉.

Safety of Acupuncture Therapies for Shoulder-hand Syndrome

Out of 62 RCTs, five studies (A67, A85, A110, A112, A114) reported information regarding the safety of acupuncture therapies. Four of them reported that no adverse events occurred. One study (A114) reported that three cases and two cases experienced subcutaneous haemorrhage in electroacupuncture group and rehabilitation group respectively. These events were mild and solved after external application.

Two of 21 non-controlled studies reported adverse events (A135, A136). Both of these studies reported one case each of feeling dizzy and nausea during acupuncture; both patients recovered after a few minutes' rest without any additional management required. Additionally, minor bleeding in the needled area was reported with six cases and eight cases, respectively, in these two studies.

Clinical Evidence for Commonly Used Acupuncture and Related Therapies

Acupuncture therapies are commonly used to manage post-stroke shoulder complications in clinical trials, and some of them are also recommended in guidelines and textbooks. Body acupuncture or electroacupuncture are the most popular treatments among the included clinical trials. In addition, some methods have been evaluated in clinical studies, but have not been recommended in clinical guidelines/textbooks; these are scalp acupuncture, floating acupuncture

浮针 and wrist-ankle acupuncture 腕踝针. The evidence of these therapies may enrich the existing clinical practice.

The most frequently reported acupuncture points are mainly those localised around the shoulder joint, such as LI15 *Jianyu* 肩髃, TE14 *Jianliao* 肩髎 and SI9 *Jianzhen* 肩贞. These acupuncture points have also been described in contemporary guidelines and textbooks (see Chapter 2).

Summary of Acupuncture and Related Therapies Clinical Evidence

Acupuncture therapies are the most common Chinese medicine treatments used in clinical practice for treating post-stroke complications. Our evaluation of clinical studies found that acupuncture therapies could improve clinically relevant outcomes of patients with post-stroke shoulder complications.

Firstly, for shoulder subluxation, there is evidence from meta-analyses supporting the benefit of adding electroacupuncture to rehabilitation in terms of improving upper limb function (FMA) and reducing pain (VAS). However, the quality of this evidence is 'low'. Also, there is evidence from single studies showing that acupuncture, electroacupuncture, scalp acupuncture and acupressure therapies had certain add-on effects when they were used in combination with rehabilitation therapy. In terms of AHI, a single study showed that adding acupressure to rehabilitation could improve treatment effect.

For post-stroke shoulder pain, clinical studies have investigated acupuncture, electroacupuncture and moxibustion as an add-on therapy to rehabilitation. Meta-analyses showed promising add-on effects for pain relief of acupuncture, moxibustion, acupuncture plus moxibustion, and floating acupuncture 浮针. In particular, the evidence of acupuncture used as an add-on therapy is of 'moderate' quality. Also, acupuncture, electroacupuncture, and acupuncture plus moxibustion have proven beneficial for upper limb function (FMA) when they were added to rehabilitation. It is noted that wrist-ankle acupuncture 腕踝针 also showed benefit on upper limb function and daily activity, but the evidence was only from a single study.

Shoulder-hand syndrome is the most commonly investigated post-stroke shoulder complication by acupuncture clinical studies. Meta-analyses support the benefit of using these as add-on therapies: acupuncture, electroacupuncture, acupuncture plus scalp acupuncture, acupuncture plus moxibustion and floating acupuncture 浮针. The add-on effects include improving upper limb function, reducing pain and improving patients' daily activities. The certainty of evidence of acupuncture and electroacupuncture is assessed as 'low' to 'moderate.' Similar to the treatment for post-stroke shoulder pain, the benefit of wrist-ankle acupuncture was shown by a single study.

Overall, few adverse events were reported, and acupuncture therapies appear to be relatively safe for the treatment of post-stroke shoulder complications. Two cases of adverse events (feeling dizzy and nausea during needling) have been reported. Such reactions might be caused by a combination of nerves or anxiety, often with not eating/drinking for quite a while before acupuncture, and possibly over-vigorous acupuncture stimulation. Acupuncture practitioners with proper training should always communicate with patients before conducting the treatment to avoid such events.

None of the studies reported the Chinese medicine syndromes. The treatment principle is inclined to select the local acupuncture points around the shoulder joint. The most frequently used acupuncture points for these three complications are LI15 *Jianyu* 肩髃, TE14 *Jianliao* 肩髎 and SI9 *Jianzhen* 肩贞. The commonly recommended acupuncture points in clinical studies are located in the Large intestine meridian 手阳明大肠经, Small intestine meridian 手太阳小肠经 and triple energizer meridian 手少阳三焦经. These points are consistent with those that may have contributed to positive effects in the meta-analyses.

In summary, acupuncture and related therapies showed promising treatment effects to improve clinical outcomes for post-stroke shoulder complications, in particular SHS. It is worth noting that there is more evidence of acupuncture and electroacupuncture than other therapies for patients with shoulder complications. The acupuncture points LI15 *Jianyu* 肩髃, TE14 *Jianliao* 肩髎 and SI9 *Jianzhen* 肩贞 should be considered as the basis of acupuncture prescription. A recently developed acupuncture technique, floating acupuncture 浮针, also could be used in combination with routine rehabilitation for treating post-stroke shoulder pain and SHS in clinical practice. The benefit of wrist-ankle acupuncture 腕踝针 is uncertain.

References

1. Lee JA, Park SW, Hwang PW, *et al.* (2012) Acupuncture for shoulder pain after stroke: A systematic review. *J Altern Complement Med* **18**(9): 818–823.
2. 聂文彬, 刘志顺, 赵宏. (2012) 针灸治疗中风后肩痛系统评价. 中国中医药信息杂志 **19**(4): 25–28.
3. 林郁芬, 李铮, 富晶晶, 刘霞. (2015) 针刺结合康复训练治疗脑卒中后肩痛的系统评价. 护士进修杂志 **30**(11): 1004–1009.
4. 卢引明, 傅立新, 牟蛟, 许红君, 祁营洲. (2009) 针灸治疗中风后肩手综合征的系统评价. *Chin J Evid-based Med* **9**(9): 976–978.
5. 徐琰, 李万瑶, 刘洁, 马林. (2013) 针灸与康复治疗脑卒中后肩手综合征疗效比较的系统评价与Meta分析. 时珍国医医药 **24**(7): 1794–1798.
6. 刘凯, 韩小蕾, 潘晓云, 熊杰. (2015) 单纯针刺治疗脑卒中后肩手综合征的系统评价. 中国康复医学杂志 **30**(10): 1041–1045.

References to Included Clinical Studies

Study No.	Reference
A1	叶斌, 白玉龙, 汪箐峰, 于健君, 徐卿, 南向亮, 孙伯平, 章伟卿. (2014) 点按肩髂穴对中风后肩关节半脱位患者的镇痛作用分析. 中医药导报 **20**(3): 22–24.
A2	李晓艳, 王艳, 黄如意. (2014) 电针结合肩部控制训练对脑卒中后肩关节半脱位的影响. 针灸临床杂志 (07): 40–42.
A3	陆瑾, 张丽霞, 刘孔江, 王彤, 陆建虎, 陈祥明, 周雪, 蒋学勇. (2010) 电针结合康复手法治疗中风后肩关节半脱位临床观察. 中国针灸 (01): 31–34.

(Continued)

(Continued)

Study No.	Reference
A4	关晨霞, 郭钢花, 李哲. (2009) 电针配合康复训练治疗脑卒中后肩关节半脱位的临床观察. 中国实用医刊 (17): 61–62.
A5	盛国滨, 卜秀焕, 龚娟娟, 周凌. (2012) 电针针刺经筋结点结合康复疗法治疗中风后肩关节半脱位的疗效观察. 针灸临床杂志 (05): 44–45.
A6	任亚平, 于青, 张志强, 李玉勤, 何磊, 陈艳红. (2012) 体针结合本体感觉神经肌肉促进技术对急性期脑卒中偏瘫患者肩关节半脱位的疗效观察. 临床和实验医学杂志 **11**(6): 407–409.
A7	杨庆红, 陈慧杰, 唐强. (2010) 头穴丛刺结合康复训练治疗脑卒中后肩关节半脱位的疗效观察. 中医药学报 **38**(6): 97–98.
A8	孟昭亮, 李晶, 王艳, 白振民. (2007) 头穴丛刺结合神经网络仪对卒中偏瘫肩关节半脱位的临床观察. 针灸临床杂志 (10): 34–35.
A9	赵一宇, 刘红玲. (2007) 头针配合康复手法治疗偏瘫肩关节半脱位. 针灸临床杂志 **23**(4): 20–21.
A10	杨年煜, 王勇丽. (2011) 针刺对中风早期肩关节半脱位的疗效观察. 河南中医 (08): 925–926.
A11	朱肖菊, 高维滨, 杨续艳. (2007) 针刺结合康复训练治疗中风后肩关节半脱位的临床观察. 北京中医药大学学报 (中医临床版) (03): 23–25.
A12	朱小娟. (2010) 针刺结合康复治疗中风后肩关节半脱位的疗效观察 [Thesis]. 南京中医药大学.
A13	胡良玉. (2014) 针刺结合康复技术治疗中风后肩关节半脱位临床疗效的观察 [Thesis]. 湖南中医药大学.
A14	张余山. (2013) 头穴丛刺结合闭链运动治疗脑卒中后肩关节半脱位的临床观察 [Thesis]. 黑龙江中医药大学.
A15	Chen CH, Chen TW, Weng MC, *et al.* (2000) The effect of electroacupuncture on shoulder subluxation for stroke patients. *Kaohsiung J Med Sci* **16**(10): 525–532.
A16	曲红伟, 王威岩, 何显峰. (2011) 针刺五输穴结合康复手法对脑卒中后肩关节半脱位的疗效观察. 中国中医药科技 **18**(1): 12.
A17	余贡献. (2012) 针灸联合运动疗法治疗脑卒中后肩关节半脱位的疗效观察. 当代医学 **18**(35): 85–86.
A18	杨来福, 王文彪, 王正辉. (2010) 电针结合康复训练治疗中风后肩关节半脱位 69 例. 中国医疗前沿 (04): 49, 54.

(Continued)

Study No.	Reference
A19	孙永. (2012) 电针透刺辅助康复治疗卒中后肩关节半脱位疗效观察. 中国伤残医学 **20**(10): 95–96.
A20	惠向联. (2014) 针灸配合电脑中频电刺激治疗中风后肩关节半脱位. 内蒙古中医药 (27): 81, 101.
A21	雷迈, 卢斌, 吴圣婕, 吴旻, 蒋瑞舟. (2009) 电针配合康复作业疗法治疗中风后肩关节半脱位60例. 广西中医药 (06): 12–13.
A22	张文娟, 龚秀琴. (2014) 艾灸结合康复护理对脑卒中后肩痛患者关节功能及生活质量的影响. 国际护理学杂志 (12): 3369–3372.
A23	潘素兰, 张冲, 邓秋兰. (2010) 艾柱灸配合康复训练治疗脑卒中偏瘫肩痛的疗效观察及护理. 辽宁中医杂志 **37**(5): 927–928.
A24	包烨华, 王延武, 楚佳梅, 朱国祥, 王翀敏, 侯海明. (2012) 电针结合康复对中风后偏瘫肩痛患者疼痛及上肢运动功能改善作用的临床观察. 中国中医药科技 **19**(1): 59–60.
A25	包烨华, 王延武, 楚佳梅, 朱国祥, 王翀敏, 侯海明. (2011) 电针结合康复对中风后偏瘫肩痛疗效观察. 中华中医药学刊 (11): 2536–2539.
A26	陆建虎, 陆瑾, 张丽霞, 刘孔江, 王彤, 陈祥明, 周雪, 蒋学勇. (2013) 电针结合康复手法治疗卒中后肩痛30例临床观察. 江苏中医药 (1): 60–61.
A27	黄丽琴. (2010) 电针配合康复治疗脑卒中偏瘫肩痛临床疗效观察. 中医药学报 **38**(4): 93–94.
A28	倪欢欢, 吴耀持, 包歆滟, 崔晓, 黄德权, 季力, 汪军, 史骏超. (2013) 浮刺配合棍棒操治疗中风后肩痛疗效观察. 上海针灸杂志 (12): 1001–1003.
A29	贺青涛, 曾科学. (2014) 浮针疗法结合康复训练治疗脑卒中后肩痛 39 例. 云南中医中药杂志 **35**(9): 56–57.
A30	陈红霞, 何铭锋, 谢仁明. (2011) 腹针结合康复训练治疗卒中后肩痛的临床观察. 南京中医药大学学报 **27**(4): 333–335.
A31	程燕玲, 李世华. (2006) 接气通经针刺法结合运动康复治疗卒中后肩痛. 针灸临床杂志 **22**(5): 39–40.
A32	刘声, 石志勇. (2013) 头针、体针配合康复训练治疗中风后偏瘫肩痛疗效观察. 世界针灸杂志 (英文版) (1): 21–26.
A33	石敦康, 唐小山. (2011) 腕踝针配合康复疗法治疗脑卒中后肩痛的临床研究. 成都中医药大学学报 **34**(1): 33–35.
A34	徐磊, 江勇, 曹小芳, 张学云, 史伟娜. (2011) 腕踝针配合康复训练治疗偏瘫肩痛. 中华全科医学 (12): 1865–1866.

(Continued)

(Continued)

Study No.	Reference
A35	肖春海, 李明. (2014) 温针灸配合康复疗法治疗中风后肩痛 22 例疗效观察. 河北中医 **36**(11): 1672–1673.
A36	郭媛媛, 陈建平. (2012) 温针治疗脑卒中后肩痛的临床研究. 中国康复医学杂志 **27**(3): 275–277.
A37	张忠霞, 张岩, 于天英, 高汉义. (2012) 针刺肩痛穴联合运动疗法治疗脑卒中偏瘫后肩痛疗效观察. 山东医药 **52**(27): 82–83.
A38	高真真, 徐道明, 李彦彩, 郭海英. (2014) 针刺结合肩部控制训练对脑卒中后肩痛的康复疗效观察. 中国康复医学杂志 **29**(4): 370–372.
A39	林奕君, 徐丽莺. (2014) 针刺结合康复训练对中风后肩痛疗效观察. 亚太传统医药 (07): 64–65.
A40	粟胜勇, 邓柏颖, 黄锦军, 胡玉英, 何育风, 黄永. (2009) 针刺治疗中风偏瘫后肩痛40例临床观察. 广西中医药 (02): 32–34.
A41	周震. (2013) 针灸联合康复治疗脑卒中后肩痛随机平行对照研究. 实用中医内科杂志 (11): 151–152.
A42	张宾. (2012) 针灸治疗偏瘫肩痛的疗效观察. 临床合理用药杂志 (15): 83.
A43	刘悦, 孙红. (2013) 针灸治疗中风后肩痛临床观察. 中国针灸 (S1): 9–10.
A44	龚辉, 唐强. (2010) 针康法治疗脑卒中后偏瘫肩痛的临床观察. 针灸临床杂志 (1): 10–11.
A45	杨继发. (2010) 腹针配合现代康复技术治疗卒中后肩痛的临床研究 [Thesis]. 广州中医药大学.
A46	陈家宏. (2013) 腹针疗法对脑卒中后肩痛患者上肢功能的影响 [Thesis]. 广州中医药大学.
A47	胡俊霞, 薛立文. (2010) 针刺结合康复训练治疗中风后肩关节疼痛 40 例. 陕西中医 **(10)**: 1392–1393.
A48	王新良, 杨延庆, 宋平. (2015) 芒针透刺配合康复治疗中风恢复期肩关节疼痛的疗效观察. 按摩与康复医学 **6**(1): 38–39.
A49	朱慎勇, 夏菊官, 王中伟. (1997) 双针巨刺治疗偏瘫性肩痛 94 例. 上海针灸杂志 (04): 28.
A50	葛俊领, 刘银鸿, 张永敏. (2007) 针推疗法治疗中风后肩痛. 四川中医 (06): 101.
A51	郭青. (2006) 滞针法电针加TDP照射治疗中风后偏瘫肩痛 50 例. 陕西中医 (07): 858–859.

(Continued)

Study No.	Reference
A52	张健. (1999) 中风肩瘫伴肩痛患者的康复治疗效果观察(附22例报告). 九江医学 (03): 148–150.
A53	张招娣, 胡蓉, 李博文, 黄选玮, 梅国胜. (2010) 腕踝针配合康复训练治疗中风偏瘫肩痛的临床疗效观察. 贵阳中医学院学报 (05): 57–58.
A54	郑盛惠, 吴玉娟, 常洁, 崔韶阳, 许明珠, 连纪伟, 魏林林. (2013) 赤凤迎源针法对脑卒中后肩手综合征患者生存质量的影响. 中医药信息 (5): 89–92.
A55	史清钊, 李春璐. (2007) 电针对缓解肩手综合征腕部水肿与疼痛疗效的观察. 航空航天医药 **18**(1): 16–18.
A56	林坚. (2008) 电针合康复训练治疗脑卒中后肩手综合征 60 例. 福建中医学院学报 **18**(3): 46–47.
A57	高鹏, 李月霞, 王志, 蒋明江, 罗郁. (2011) 电针及康复训练对肩手综合征的疗效分析. 按摩与康复医学 **2**(2): 49–50.
A58	段英春, 刘芳, 张彦. (2014) 电针结合康复训练治疗肩手综合征. 吉林中医药 (2): 190–191.
A59	乔桂芳, 郑威平. (2012) 电针结合气压循环治疗脑卒中后肩手综合征临床观察. 按摩与康复医学 **3**(33): 401–402.
A60	黎明全. (2013) 电针手阳明经五腧穴治疗脑卒中后肩手综合征临床研究. 吉林中医药 (2): 191–192.
A61	汪军, 崔晓, 倪欢欢, 黄春水, 周翠侠, 吴佶, 史骏超, 吴毅. (2013) 浮刺合康复训练治疗脑卒中后肩手综合征肩部疼痛疗效观察. 中国针灸 **33**(4): 294–298.
A62	倪欢欢, 崔晓, 胡永善, 冯美兰, 周翠侠, 史骏超. (2010) 浮刺结合功能训练治疗肩手综合征疗效观察. 上海针灸杂志 **29**(6): 367–368.
A63	王翀敏, 陈晓禹. (2011) 浮针疗法结合康复训练治疗卒中后肩手综合征 30 例临床观察. 江苏中医药 **43**(3): 67–68.
A64	杨丹, 何晓晓, 蔡伟, 杨孝芳, 杨梅. (2015) 浮针配合康复治疗卒中后肩手综合征疗效观察及机制探讨. 时珍国医国药 **26**(1): 139–141.
A65	杜何欣, 杜雪峰, 杨路庭, 董正军, 景兰芳. (2012) 隔附子饼灸治疗脑卒中后肩手综合征临床观察. 中国中医药信息杂志 (01): 71–72.
A66	张铭, 黄莹. (2011) 红外线穴位照射治疗中风后肩手综合征的临床分析. 中国实用神经疾病杂志 (24): 60–61.
A67	徐世芬, 庄礼兴, 贾超, 许德敬, 潘超安. (2010) 靳三针疗法配合功能训练治疗中风偏瘫后肩手综合征的临床观察. 广州中医药大学学报 (1): 19–22.

(Continued)

Study No.	Reference
A68	林涵, 庄礼兴, 贺君. (2012) 靳三针疗法治疗卒中后肩手综合征随机对照研究. 广州中医药大学学报 **29**(4): 389–391, 401.
A69	武峙璇, 金泽. (2011) 颈部央脊穴结合透刺针法治疗中风肩手综合征60例临床观察. 黑龙江中医药 **40**(5): 51.
A70	侯智. (2014) 康复训练结合针灸治疗脑卒中后肩手综合征Ⅰ期的疗效评价. 实用临床医药杂志 **18**(5): 58–59, 66.
A71	贾澄杰, 倪光夏, 谭辉, 张娴. (2012) 康复训练结合针灸治疗脑卒中后肩手综合征Ⅰ期临床疗效观察. 长春中医药大学学报 **28**(4): 711–712.
A72	周飞雄, 曾科学, 陆彦青. (2013) 康复训练配合太极针法治疗卒中后肩手综合征临床疗效观察. 现代诊断与治疗 **24**(5): 1004–1006.
A73	常文艳, 杨欣. (2013) 雷火灸结合康复手法治疗肩手综合征临床观察. 辽宁中医药大学学报 **15**(9): 191–192.
A74	刘远明. (2009) 缪刺肩痛穴结合康复训练治疗肩手综合征的临床研究. 甘肃医药 **28**(3): 176–178.
A75	林志瑜. (2008) 缪刺条口结合康复训练治疗肩手综合征的临床研究. 中国社区医师•医学专业 **10**(23): 150–151.
A76	李岚, 马臣, 崔旻, 王晓芳, 李丽娜, 韩广云. (2011) 脑卒中后肩手综合征康复治疗临床观察. 按摩与康复医学 **2**(14): 92.
A77	苏久龙, 潘翠环, 万新炉. (2010) 平衡针刺及功能训练治疗脑卒中后肩手综合征. 中国康复 **25**(3): 188–189.
A78	李念. (2014) 平衡针刺及康复训练治疗脑卒中后肩手综合征临床观察. 四川中医 **32**(4): 161–162.
A79	万新炉, 苏久龙, 叶正茂, 罗仁浩, 曾永媚. (2012) 平衡针刺结合功能训练对脑卒中后肩手综合征的疗效观察. 国际医药卫生导报 **18**(24): 3534–3537.
A80	尹景春. (2014) 全经针刺结合康复训练治疗中风后肩手综合征的临床观察 [Thesis]. 湖南中医药大学.
A81	徐海燕, 熊俊, 何立东. (2014) 热敏灸结合针刺治疗脑卒中后肩手综合征Ⅰ期临床观察. 亚太传统医药 **10**(19): 96–98.
A82	温静, 张连城. (2009) 调神通络法结合康复训练治疗卒中后肩手综合征 30 例临床观察. 江苏中医药 (8): 55–56.
A83	秦宏, 施丽俊, 张宇, 马丹, 高强. (2013) 头穴透刺配合康复训练治疗脑卒中后肩手综合征疗效观察. 上海针灸杂志 **32**(3): 167–169.

(Continued)

(Continued)

Study No.	Reference
A84	冯玲媚, 刘明辉. (2012) 腕踝针结合康复训练治疗脑梗死后肩手综合征的临床疗效观察. 辽宁中医杂志 **39**(6): 1147–1148.
A85	聂文彬, 赵宏. (2011) 温通三焦法配合康复训练治疗肩手综合征临床观察. 上海针灸杂志 **30**(4): 217–219.
A86	邱昌民. (2011) 温针灸结合康复疗法治疗脑卒中后肩手综合征临床观察. 中国中医急症 **20**(5): 699, 736.
A87	刘志文, 费英俊, 郜时华, 钱蕾. (2013) 温针灸结合运动疗法治疗脑卒中后肩手综合征的疗效观察. 中国疗养医学 **22**(2): 139–140.
A88	史术峰. (2012) 循经远端选穴配合运动疗法治疗肩手综合征. 针灸临床杂志 **28**(5): 18–20.
A89	吴志刚. (2014) 针刺结合康复训练治疗脑卒中后肩手综合征 100 例. 中国中医药现代远程教育 (20): 81–82.
A90	杨健. (2011) 针刺结合康复训练治疗脑卒中后肩手综合征 43 例疗效观察. 河北中医药学报 **26**(1): 27–28.
A91	尚艳杰, 马程程, 蔡玉颖, 王东升, 孔令丽. (2008) 针刺结合康复治疗中风后肩手综合征. 中国针灸 (05): 331–333.
A92	万文蓉, 王天磊, 程绍鲁, 赵银龙, 张卫, 吴秋燕, 金海鹏, 洪秀瑜, 李应霞. (2013) 针刺结合康复治疗中风后肩手综合征:随机对照研究. 中国针灸 **33**(11): 970–974.
A93	赵素萍. (2014) 针刺联合康复训练治疗脑卒中后肩手综合征 40 例. 河南中医 **34**(9): 1823–1825.
A94	林红霞, 叶关泉, 廖辉雄, 林方毅, 梁碧君. (2014) 针刺联合康复训练治疗脑卒中后肩手综合征的疗效观察. 世界中医药 (1): 84–85, 88.
A95	陈静. (2014) 针刺联合神经妥乐平治疗脑卒中后肩手综合征 30 例疗效观察. 湖南中医杂志 (7): 101–102.
A96	王小清, 高崇, 马松武. (2012) 针刺配合康复训练治疗脑卒中后肩手综合征的疗效观察. 临床和实验医学杂志 **11**(12): 942–943.
A97	于春梅, 毛忠南. (2011) 针刺配合手法康复治疗肩手综合征 (Ⅰ期) 60 例疗效观察. 中国社区医师 **27**(40): 16.
A98	滕秀英, 王杨. (2012) 针刺人迎穴为主治疗脑梗死后肩手综合征临床观察. 上海针灸杂志 **31**(8): 562–563.
A99	陈鸣. (2008) 针刺治疗脑卒中后肩手综合症的临床观察. 中国热带医学 **8**(10): 1717, 1781.

(Continued)

(Continued)

Study No.	Reference
A100	汤治中, 徐应乐, 易进科, 王文科, 汤勇. (2013) 针灸结合康复训练对肩手综合征患者肩痛及运动功能的影响. 陕西中医 (7): 882–883.
A101	沈振华. (2014) 针灸结合康复训练治疗肩手综合征疗效观察. 深圳中西医结合杂志 (08): 56–58.
A102	杨秋汇, 吕福全. (2011) 中西医结合治疗中风后肩手综合征临床观察. 黑龙江中医药 (05): 45–46.
A103	钟青, 冯琼华, 易刚. (2011) 综合康复疗法治疗脑卒中后肩手综合征的疗效观察. 实用医院临床杂志 **8**(4): 115–116.
A104	冯晓东. (2008) 综合疗法对脑卒中后肩手综合征患者 60 例临床疗效观察. 中国实用神经疾病杂志 **11**(4): 76–77.
A105	章荣, 周蜜娟. (2008) 综合疗法治疗卒中后肩手综合征疗效观察. 中国康复医学杂志 **23**(6): 545–546.
A106	廖华薇. (2006) 作业疗法合针灸治疗肩手综合征45例疗效观察. 上海针灸杂志 (03): 9–10.
A107	李峰, 涂美. (2013) 作业疗法配合电针治疗 脑卒中后肩手综合征 I 期疗效观察. 中国药物经济学 (S3): 370–371.
A108	郑盛惠, 吴玉娟, 常洁, 崔韶阳, 许明珠, 连纪伟, 魏林林. (2013) 赤凤迎源针法治疗脑卒中后肩手综合征的疗效观察. 中国康复 (1): 40–41.
A109	邱婷婷. (2011) 针刺结合运动疗法治疗脑卒中后肩手综合征的临床研究 [Thesis]. 黑龙江中医药大学.
A110	谢芹. (2010) 针刺结合康复训练治疗脑卒中肩手综合征的临床研究 [Thesis]. 广州中医药大学.
A111	宋祖琪. (2011) 电针与低频电治疗中风后肩手综合征疗效的比较研究 [Thesis]. 湖北中医药大学.
A112	徐哲. (2008) 电针手阳明经五输穴治疗中风后肩手综合征的临床观察 [Thesis]. 长春中医药大学.
A113	尤阳. (2011) 电针配合康复训练治疗脑卒中后肩手综合征的临床研究 [Thesis]. 山东中医药大学.
A114	张效玮. (2011) 电针结合康复训练治疗中风后肩手综合征的疗效观察 [Thesis]. 广州中医药大学.
A115	武峭璇. (2011) 颈部夹脊穴结合透刺针法治疗卒中后肩手综合征 I 期的临床疗效 [Thesis]. 黑龙江中医药大学.

(Continued)

Study No.	Reference
A116	程小平. (2008) [Treatment of 40 Cases of Post-stroke Shoulder-Hand Syndrome by Acupuncture.] 针灸推拿医学 (英文版) **6**(1): 17–18.
A117	朱永刚, 苏清伦, 赵秦, 王慧海. (2011) 电针结合艾灸治疗中风后肩手综合征 30 例. 广西中医药 (06): 25–26.
A118	陈毕能,付谦,李莉. (2012) 电针结合康复训练治疗肩手综合征 96 例分析. 中国误诊学杂志 **12**(17): 4682.
A119	杨来福,郭学军. (2009)电针与综合康复治疗脑卒中后肩手综合征 54 例. 医学信息 (10): 2088–2090.
A120	段英春,刘芳,杨晓禹. (2014) 电针治疗脑卒中后肩手综合征 36 例. 吉林中医药 (4): 415–416.
A121	刘刚,林妙君. (2012) 电致孔脉冲仪配合正清风痛宁透药治疗中风后肩手综合征 30 例临床观察. 中医药导报 **18**(4): 98–99.
A122	周昭辉,庄礼兴,江钢辉,李艳慧,徐展琼,廖穆熙,何冠蘅. (2014) 浮针疗法治疗中风后肩手综合征临床观察. 针灸临床杂志 (02): 28–30.
A123	杨思奇. (2011) 热敏灸配合康复训练治疗脑卒中后肩手综合征 46 例. 吉林中医药 **31**(9): 887–888.
A124	冯宝领,郑健刚. (2012) 醒脑开窍针刺加康复训练治疗脑卒中后肩手综合征 42 例疗效观察. 黑龙江中医药 (01): 33–34.
A125	邢丹智,金明珠,王小琴. (2008) 针刺关节松动术治疗脑卒中病后肩手综合征 14 例疗效观察. 中国民康医学 **20**(5A): 932–933.
A126	沙碧源, 尹昌浩, 赵维纳. (2010) 针刺配合手法康复治疗脑中风后肩-手综合征 46 例临床观察. 实用心脑肺血管病杂志 **18**(4): 471.
A127	李杰. (2006) 针刺为主治疗中风后肩手综合征的临床体会. 四川中医 (09): 106–107.
A128	刘运珠,张美花. (2007) 针刺运动疗法治疗脑卒中并发肩手综合征 60 例. 江苏中医药 **39**(9): 54.
A129	蔡超群. (2002) 中药穴位烫疗脑卒中后肩手综合征的观察及护理 40 例. 实用护理杂志 (07): 53.
A130	石翠霞,谢瑞娟,王晓红,杨艳玲,邓赟,陈璐. (2013) 综合康复疗法治疗脑卒中后肩手综合征. 医学研究与教育 **30**(6): 65–67, 85.
A131	张建宏,范建中,彭楠,齐志强. (2005) 综合康复治疗脑卒中后肩手综合征的疗效观察. 中华物理医学与康复杂志 **27**(9): 537–540.

(Continued)

(*Continued*)

Study No.	Reference
A132	甘惠珍. (2009) 综合治疗脑血管病肩手综合徵的疗效观察. 华夏医药 **4**(5): 387–388.
A133	郑婕,朱现民. (2014) 隔姜泥重灸法治疗卒中后肩手综合征的临床体会. 中国民间疗法 (12): 11–12.
A134	谢芹,庄礼兴,贺君. (2011) 靳三针治疗脑卒中后肩手综合征疗效观察. 上海针灸杂志 (07): 462–463.
A135	顾宝光. (2009) 长圆针治疗偏瘫后肩手综合征 I 期临床疗效及安全性观察 [Thesis]. 北京中医药大学.
A136	梁翠梅. (2010) 长圆针治疗脑卒中偏瘫后肩手综合征 I 期疗效观察 [Thesis]. 北京中医药大学.

8

Post-stroke Shoulder Complications: Clinical Evidence for Other Chinese Medicine Therapies

OVERVIEW

Along with Chinese herbal medicine and acupuncture therapies, other Chinese medicine therapies, such as traditional Chinese *tuina* 推拿 or cupping therapy, can be used clinically to treat post-stroke shoulder complications. This chapter provides a synopsis of the clinical trial literature and an assessment of the state of evidence. Extensive searches were undertaken in nine English and Chinese databases, and identified citations were assessed against inclusion criteria. Eleven randomised controlled trials were selected for inclusion in this chapter, and were subject to systematic review and evaluation of their efficacy and safety. There is limited evidence available for other Chinese medicine therapies for post-stroke shoulder complications.

Introduction

In addition to Chinese herbal medicine (CHM) and acupuncture therapies, Chinese medicine (CM) includes a range of other therapies to treat disease and maintain health. These include:

- Traditional Chinese *tuina* 推拿: Chinese massage therapy;
- Cupping therapy: Application of suction by placing a vacuumised cup onto the body.

This chapter evaluates the clinical evidence of other CM therapies for the post-stroke shoulder complications including: (1) shoulder subluxation; (2) shoulder pain and (3) shoulder-hand syndrome. Data from randomised controlled trials (RCTs) were evaluated for efficacy and safety. Non-controlled clinical studies were summarised for key information of relevant treatments.

Identification of Clinical Studies

A total of 37,141 citations was identified after searching Chinese and English databases. At the end, 11 RCTs (O1–O11) and four non-controlled clinical studies (O12–O15) were included according to the inclusion criteria (Fig. 8.1). *Tuina* 推拿 therapy was used in nine RCTs and four non-controlled studies, and cupping therapy was used in two RCTs.

Of the 11 RCTs, one study (O1) investigated shoulder subluxation and shoulder pain, two studies (O2, O3) focused on shoulder subluxation, four studies (O4–O7) were of shoulder pain, and the other four studies (O8–O11) focused on shoulder-hand syndrome (SHS). All RCTs were conducted in mainland China with a total of 784 participants being involved. The age of participants ranged from 28 years (O1) to 79 years (O4). Of the studies that reported clear information on participants' gender, there were more males ($n = 421$) than females ($n = 283$).

Among the four non-controlled studies, one study was for shoulder subluxation (O14), one study was for general post-stroke shoulder complications (O15), and the other two targeted SHS (O12, O13). All these studies investigated the *tuina* 推拿 therapy, with a total of 271 participants being involved in these studies (O12–O15).

In addition, eight studies were identified using intervention not commonly practised outside of China; they will not be presented in this chapter.

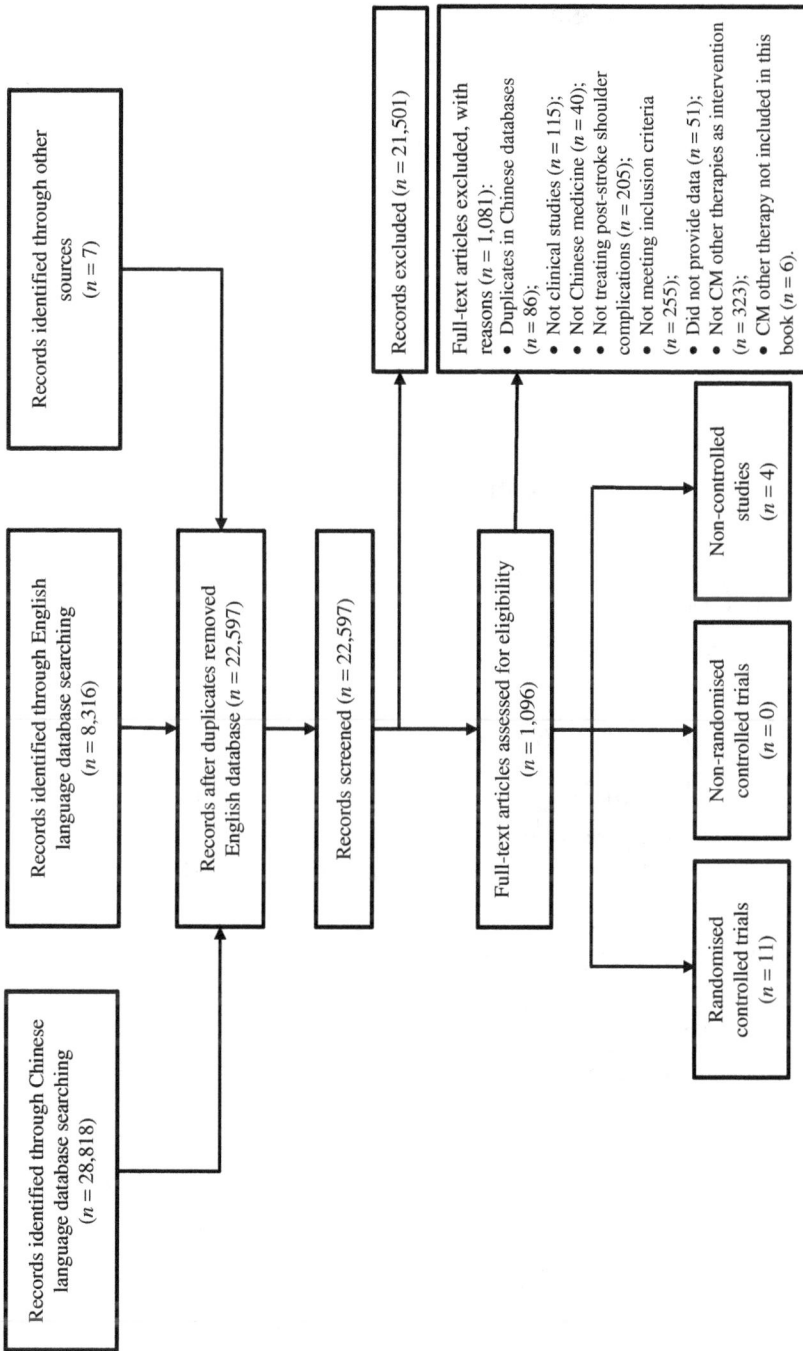

Fig. 8.1 Flowchart of study selection process: Other Chinese medicine therapies for post-stroke shoulder complications.

Risk of Bias Assessment of Included Randomised Controlled Trials

All included studies were described as RCTs. However, seven studies did not report the details of the methods for randomisation sequence generation and were judged as 'unclear' risk for this domain. In addition, four studies applied incorrect randomisation methods, and were therefore judged as 'high' risk. All studies were 'unclear' risk for allocation concealment due to lack of information. Blinding of participants and personnel was judged as 'high' risk of bias in all studies because they were all designed to evaluate add-on effects without any effort of blinding. Blinding of outcome assessors were all 'unclear' risk due to lack of information. Incomplete outcome data was assessed as 'low' risk of bias for all studies. All studies were assessed 'unclear' risk for selective reporting as protocols or trial registration could not be identified for the studies. Overall the methodological quality was 'low'; results should be interpreted with caution. See Table 8.1 for a summary.

Shoulder Subluxation

Shoulder subluxation is a common complication of stroke. Management of post-stroke shoulder subluxation aims at reducing pain and preventing it from worsening. Chinese medicine therapy,

Table 8.1 Risk of Bias Assessment of Randomised Controlled Trials

Risk of Bias Domain	Low Risk *n* (%)	Unclear Risk *n* (%)	High Risk *n* (%)
Sequence generation	0	7 (63.4)	4 (27.3)
Allocation concealment	0	11 (100)	0
Blinding of participants	0	0	11 (100)
Blinding of personnel	0	0	11 (100)
Blinding of outcome assessors	0	11 (100)	0
Incomplete outcome data	11 (100)	0	0
Selective outcome reporting	0	11 (100)	0

e.g. *tuina* 推拿 around the shoulder joint could assist strengthening local muscles and pain relief.

Three RCTs (O1–O3) and one non-controlled clinical study (O14) were found evaluating the combination of *tuina* 推拿 and rehabilitation for managing subluxation. These four studies were conducted in China and published between 2012 and 2015.

Randomised Controlled Trials of *Tuina* 推拿 Therapy

Three RCTs (O1–O3) involving 190 participants (male 123, female 67) were included in our evaluation. All these three studies evaluated the combination of *tuina* 推拿 and rehabilitation for managing subluxation. The duration of disease ranged from three weeks to nine months (O3).

One RCT (O2) compared the combination of *tuina* 推拿 and rehabilitation to rehabilitation alone on 100 participants with post-stroke shoulder subluxation. *Tuina* 推拿 therapy was performed by the clinician on shoulder muscles (deltoid, trapezius, supraspinatus and infraspinatus) and acupuncture points (LI15 *Jianyu* 肩髃, SI9 *Jianzhen* 肩贞, GB21 *Jianjing* 肩井 and SI11 *Tianzong* 天宗). This treatment was applied for 50 minutes in each session, five times a week for six weeks continually. Using Fugl-Meyer Assessment (FMA) as an outcome measure, it was found that the combination of *tuina* 推拿 and rehabilitation achieved greater treatment effect than rehabilitation alone (MD: 7.18, [2.64, 11.72]). This study also measured the acromiohumeral interval (AHI) (from the cortical bone at the inferior aspect of the acromion to the humeral head) to determine the severity of shoulder joint subluxation. It was found that the combined treatment achieved better effect for this outcome (MD: −2.16 [−3.88, −0.44]). One RCT (O1) measured FMA, pain visual analogue scale (VAS) and AHI but detailed data was not reported.

In addition, effective rate data was reported by all three studies (O1–O3). However, the results were not pooled for the meta-analysis because the criteria for assessing effective rate were not consistent.

Non-controlled Clinical Studies of *Tuina* 推拿 Therapy

One non-controlled clinical study (O14) was found using the combination of *tuina* 推拿 and rehabilitation for managing post-stroke shoulder subluxation. *Tuina* 推拿 therapy was applied focusing on local acupuncture points and then on local muscles. Reduction in shoulder joint dislocation was required at the end of each treatment session.

Shoulder Pain

Following subluxation, sufferers can experience pain requiring clinical intervention to reduce the pain and improve the range of motion to the shoulder. Five RCTs (O1, O4–O7) involving 358 participants were identified from the search which evaluated treatment effects on post-stroke shoulder pain. These five studies investigated the add-on effects of CM therapies, with four studies (O1, O4–O6) comparing the combination of *tuina* 推拿 and rehabilitation to rehabilitation alone, and one RCT (O7) evaluating the combination of cupping therapy and rehabilitation. The treatment duration ranged from three weeks (O4) to eight weeks (O1).

There were no non-randomised controlled or non-controlled studies found that focused on post-stroke shoulder pain.

Randomised Controlled Trials of *Tuina* 推拿 Therapy

Four RCTs compared the combination of *tuina* 推拿 and routine care/rehabilitation to rehabilitation alone (O1, O4–O6). Outcomes reported by these four studies included FMA score, pain VAS, range of motion (ROM) and effective rate.

Fugl-Meyer Assessment (Upper Limb)

One study (O4) reported data on upper limb FMA outcome measure. It was found that the combination was superior to routine care and rehabilitation (MD: 6.00 [3.85, 8.15]).

Pain Visual Analogue Scale

Three RCTs (O4–O6), including a total of 244 participants, reported data on pain VAS. The Zhong study (O5) used a 100-point VAS while the other two studies all used a 10-point VAS for assessing pain. After converting the data of Zhong (O5), meta-analyses of four studies showed that the combination was more effective for reducing pain than rehabilitation alone (MD: –1.05 [–1.69, –0.42], $I^2 = 84\%$).

Range of Motion

One RCT (O4) reported data on the range of motion of shoulder joint lifting. The results showed that the combined therapy was more effective than routine rehabilitation for promoting shoulder movement (MD: 23.30 [21.43, 25.17]).

Effective Rate

Two RCTs (O1, O6) reported data of effective rate. Data were not pooled for analysis due to the unclear method of calculation.

Assessment Using GRADE

A summary of findings table was prepared for the comparisons of *tuina* 推拿 therapy plus rehabilitation vs. rehabilitation alone (Table 8.2). The evidence of benefit of adding *tuina* 推拿 therapy to rehabilitation for FMA and shoulder ROM was assessed as 'low' certainty, while the evidence of that for pain VAS was 'very low' certainty.

Randomised Controlled Trials of Cupping Therapy

One RCT (O7) compared the combination of mobile cupping therapy with rehabilitation to rehabilitation alone. Cupping was applied on the painful area during shoulder movement. Using upper limb FMA as the outcome measure, it was found that combination therapy

Table 8.2 *Tuina* 推拿 Therapy Plus Rehabilitation vs. Rehabilitation Alone for Shoulder Pain

Outcomes	No. of Participants (Studies) Follow-up	Certainty of the Evidence (GRADE)	Risk with Rehabilitation	Anticipated Absolute Effects	
				Risk Difference with *Tuina* 推拿 + Rehabilitation	
FMA	80 (1 RCT)	⊕⊕◯◯ LOW[a,b]	The mean FMA was **15.7** points	MD **6 points higher** (3.85 higher to 8.15 higher)	
Pain VAS	244 (3 RCTs)	⊕◯◯◯ VERY LOW[a,b,c]	The mean VAS was **3.75** points	MD **1.05 points lower** (1.69 lower to 0.42 lower)	
Shoulder range of motion	80 (1 RCT)	⊕⊕◯◯ LOW[a,b]	The mean shoulder range of motion was **145.5 degrees**	MD **23.3 degrees higher** (21.43 higher to 25.17 higher)	

The risk in the intervention group (and its 95% confidence interval) is based on the assumed risk in the comparison group and the relative effect of the intervention (and its 95% CI).

Abbreviations: CI, confidence interval; FMA, Fugl-Meyer Assessment; GRADE, Grading of Recommendations Assessment, Development and Evaluation; MD, mean difference; RCT, randomised control trial; VAS, visual analogue scale.

Notes:

a. Lack of blinding of participants, personnel and assessors;
b. Small sample size limits certainty of results;
c. Considerable statistical heterogeneity.

Study Reference:

FMA: O4
Pain VAS: O4–O6
Shoulder range of motion: O4

achieved significant superior effects (MD: 3.98 [2.53, 5.43]). This study also reported numeric rating scale (NRS) to assess the pain severity. Using NRS, it was found that the combination of cupping and rehabilitation was more effective than rehabilitation alone (MD: −2.01 [−2.73, −1.29]).

Shoulder-hand Syndrome

The treatment goals of SHS are reducing pain, maintaining joint mobility and restoring shoulder function. Chinese medicine therapies may assist routine care to eliminate pain and swelling, as well as to improve the shoulder function.

Four RCTs (O8–O11), involving 286 participants, were identified that investigated SHS. All these studies investigated the add-on effects of CM therapies, with three of these (O9–O11) comparing the combination of *tuina* 推拿 and rehabilitation to rehabilitation alone, and another one (O8) comparing the combination of cupping therapy and rehabilitation to rehabilitation alone. The treatment duration was only reported in one RCT (O11) and ranged from 16 days to 180 days.

Two non-controlled clinical studies (O12–O13) using the combination of *tuina* 推拿 and routine rehabilitation for the management of SHS were found.

Randomised Controlled Trials of *Tuina* 推拿 Therapy

Three RCTs (O9–O11) compared the combination of *tuina* 推拿 and rehabilitation to rehabilitation alone. Treatment effects are presented below under each outcome.

Fugl-Meyer Assessment

Upper limb FMA score was reported by two studies (O9–O10), involving a total of 140 participants. Meta-analysis showed no statistically significant difference between the combined therapy and rehabilitation for upper limb FMA scores (MD: 5.89 [−1.34, 13.11], $I^2 = 96\%$). High heterogeneity of these two studies was detected.

Pain Visual Analogue Scale

Pain is one of the major symptoms of SHS. Using a 100-point VAS to assess pain, one study of 60 participants (O10) reported that the pain score of both groups decreased after 45 days of treatment; however, there was no statistically significant difference between the combined therapy and rehabilitation alone (MD: −1.48 [−4.25, 1.29]).

Activities of Daily Living

One study involving 80 participants (O9) reported data on activities of daily living (ADL). For this outcome, the combination of *tuina* 推拿 and rehabilitation was more effective than rehabilitation alone (MD: 20.22 [14.15, 26.29]).

Effective Rate

Two studies (O9, O11) reported data on effective rate. These data were not pooled for a meta-analysis due to the unclear methods of effective rate calculation.

Assessment Using GRADE

A summary of findings table was prepared for the comparisons of *tuina* 推拿 therapy plus rehabilitation vs. rehabilitation alone (Table 8.3). The evidence of benefit of adding *tuina* 推拿 therapy to rehabilitation for FMA and pain VAS was assessed as 'very low' certainty, while the evidence of that for ADL was 'low' certainty.

Non-Controlled Clinical Studies of *Tuina* 推拿 Therapy

Two non-controlled clinical studies (O12, O13) evaluated the combination of *tuina* 推拿 and routine rehabilitation for SHS. A total of 124 participants was involved in these studies. *Tuina* 推拿 was applied on the shoulder, arm and hand, aiming to reduce pain and swelling, as well as to improve the range of movement.

Table 8.3 *Tuina* 推拿 Therapy Plus Rehabilitation vs. Rehabilitation for Shoulder-hand Syndrome

Outcomes	No. of Participants (Studies) Follow-up	Certainty of the Evidence (GRADE)	Anticipated Absolute Effects	
			Risk with Rehabilitation	Risk Difference with *Tuina* 推拿 + Rehabilitation
FMA	140 (2 RCTs)	⊕◯◯◯ VERY LOW[a,b,c]	The mean FMA was **43.18** points	MD **5.89 points higher** (1.34 lower to 13.11 higher)
VAS	60 (1 RCT)	⊕◯◯◯ VERY LOW[a,c]	The mean VAS was **43.25** points	MD **1.48 points lower** (4.25 lower to 1.29 higher)
ADL	80 (1 RCT)	⊕⊕◯◯ LOW[a,d]	The mean ADL was **52.74** points	MD **20.22 points higher** (14.15 higher to 26.29 higher)

The risk in the intervention group (and its 95% confidence interval) is based on the assumed risk in the comparison group and the relative effect of the intervention (and its 95% CI).

Abbreviations: ADL, activities of daily living; CI, confidence interval; FMA, Fugl-Meyer Assessment; GRADE, Grading of Recommendations Assessment, Development and Evaluation; MD, mean difference; RCT, randomised control trial; VAS, visual analogue scale.

Notes:

a. Lack of blinding of participants, personnel and assessors;
b. Considerable statistical heterogeneity;
c. Small sample size limits certainty of results and 95% CI overlaps no effect;
d. Small sample size limits certainty of results

Study Reference:

FMA: O9,O10
VAS: O10
ADL: O9

Randomised Controlled Trials of Cupping Therapy

One RCT (O8) combined flash cupping therapy with routine rehabilitation for the treatment of SHS. Cupping therapy was applied on
acupuncture points around the shoulder joint (LI15 *Jianyu* 肩髃, SI9
Jianzhen 肩贞, TE14 *Jianliao* 肩髎 and SI11 *Tianzong* 天宗). This study
concluded that combining cupping therapy with rehabilitation was
more effective than routine rehabilitation alone. However, the treatment effects could not be confirmed because the only outcome
reported was effective rate.

Safety of Other Chinese Medicine Therapies

Nine RCTs and four non-controlled clinical studies evaluated *tuina*
推拿; of these, only one non-controlled clinical study (O13) mentioned that no adverse events occurred. None of the other studies
reported information on adverse events.

Two RCTs (O7, O8) investigated adding cupping therapy to routine rehabilitation for managing post-stroke shoulder pain. Neither
study reported information on adverse events.

Evidence for Other Chinese Medicine Therapies Commonly Used in Clinical Practice

Tuina 推拿 therapy has been recommended by a clinical guideline
for the treatment of post-stroke shoulder complications (see Chapter 2).
It is recommended that *tuina* 推拿 therapy be applied on the acupuncture points around the shoulder joint; however, strong stimulation
of the spasm muscle should be avoided.

Our review of clinical studies found that *tuina* 推拿 therapy had
been evaluated by a group of clinical studies. There is promising
evidence from RCTs supporting the use of *tuina* 推拿 therapy as add-
on therapy for all three types of shoulder complications. For example,
for shoulder subluxation, adding *tuina* 推拿 therapy could assist in
reducing AHI and improving patients' upper limb function. For people who suffer from shoulder pain, it is effective in pain management

and improves shoulder movement as well as upper limb function. Once SHS has developed, using *tuina* 推拿 therapy is beneficial for improving patients' daily activities.

Tuina 推拿 therapy is usually applied on the local shoulder muscles and acupuncture points, which is consistent with clinical guideline recommendations (see Chapter 2). It is important to note that, when performing *tuina* 推拿 therapy, strong stimulation should be avoided to prevent potential injury of the joint capsule.

Summary of Clinical Evidence for Other Chinese Medicine Therapies

Our review of clinical studies found that *tuina* 推拿 therapy used as an add-on therapy to routine rehabilitation is beneficial for upper limb function (FMA), shoulder joint ROM (lifting) and pain symptoms of shoulder subluxation and pain. The evidence of *tuina* 推拿 therapy when used as an add-on therapy is assessed as 'very low' to 'low' quality. For SHS, the current evidence showed that adding *tuina* 推拿 therapy to routine rehabilitation could improve patients' daily activity; however, it may not be beneficial for relieving pain and improving upper limb function. This might be due to the fact that there are only a very small number of studies with limited participants involved. The certainty of such evidence is also 'very low' to 'low'. On the other hand, *tuina* 推拿 therapy seems safe in clinical practice as long as it is performed following certain protocols. It has been pointed out by multiple studies that strong stimulation should be avoided during *tuina* 推拿 therapy.

Tuina 推拿 therapy could be conducted daily for 30–40 minutes each time. Chinese medicine syndrome differentiation is not essential for the *tuina* 推拿 therapy. Affected muscles should be identified before the *tuina* 推拿 therapy begins. Acupuncture points around the shoulder joint are also often selected during *tuina* 推拿 therapy.

Furthermore, cupping therapy proved effective when used as an add-on therapy for shoulder pain. Mobile cupping on the painful area during shoulder movement could reduce pain symptoms and improve upper limb function. However, whether using flash cupping on the acupuncture points around the shoulder joint is beneficial for SHS has not been confirmed. Although the two studies presented did not report any adverse events caused by cupping, it is important to note that applying cupping on post-stroke patients may cause unwanted adverse events due to the patients' decreased sensation.

In terms of the outcome measures, pain score (VAS or NRS) was most commonly reported. In fact, the shoulder complications are not only related to pain. More importantly, they are closely related to upper limb function and therefore, affect patients' daily activities. As a result, FMA and ADL should also be assessed by these studies. In addition, only one study for shoulder subluxation reported data on AHI, which specifically measures the shoulder joint pathologies.

As no minimal clinically important difference has been determined for the outcomes in post-stroke shoulder complications, the clinical relevance of these findings remains uncertain. Similar to the CHM clinical evidence, the time of starting these therapies was not consistently reported by the included clinical studies. Further research may consider taking this into consideration.

References to Included Clinical Studies

Study No.	References
O1	张昕煜, 徐寅平. (2015) 整合按摩手法结合现代康复技术治疗中风后肩痛伴肩关节半脱位25例. 中国中医药现代远程教育 (5): 74–76.
O2	叶斌, 白玉龙, 孙莉敏, 汪箐峰, 徐卿, 南向亮, 周磊, 徐国琴. (2014) 按揉结合治疗中风后肩关节半脱位的临床疗效分析. 医学临床研究 (1): 26–27, 30.
O3	赵英子, 何丹, 穆青, 李萌. (2013) 推拿手法在肩关节半脱位综合康复治疗中应用效果的临床观察. 航空航天医学杂志 (6): 650–651.
O4	汪强, 李杰. (2011) 康复训练加推拿治疗脑卒中后偏瘫肩痛疗效观察. 按摩与康复医学 (12): 102–103.
O5	钟杰, 鲁凤琴, 苏扬. (2004) 脑卒中偏瘫肩痛的康复治疗. 中国社区医师(综合版) (15): 62–63.
O6	杨波, 邢雪梅, 刘佳, 张秀峰. (2014) 推拿结合康复治疗中风偏瘫肩痛的疗效观察. 贵阳中医学院学报 (3): 135–138.

(Continued)

(Continued)

Study No.	References
O7	杨梅云. (2013) 康复训练结合拔罐治疗脑卒中后肩痛64例疗效观察. 国医论坛 (6): 26–27.
O8	程学莲, 程春霞. (2014) 拔罐联合常规对症及康复训练治疗中风后肩手综合征随机平行对照研究. 实用中医内科杂志 (11): 27–29.
O9	朱永刚, 苏清纶, 赵秦. (2011) 推拿结合康复训练治疗脑卒中后肩手综合征80例临床观察. 按摩与康复医学 (10): 16–17.
O10	刘旸, 郭雪梅, 刘先虎, 翁浩. (2011) 推拿配合肩胛控制训练治疗偏瘫患者肩手综合征的疗效观察. 现代中西医结合杂志 (19): 2347–2349.
O11	石新. (2011) 平乐郭氏荣肌揉筋法结合康复训练治疗肩手综合征疗效观察. 山西中医 (7): 30–31.
O12	卫其华. (2008) 手法结合理疗治疗脑卒中后肩手综合征32例疗效观察. 按摩与导引 (3): 29–30.
O13	夏振君, 李旭华. (2013) 推拿肩部、手部、前臂肌肉联合温热磁振治疗脑卒中后肩-手综合征 92 例临床观察. 实用中医内科杂志 (5): 132–133.
O14	袁洪雷, 李计, 韩峰. (2012) 推拿手法治疗脑卒中后肩关节半脱位疗效观察. 中国中医药信息杂志 (7): 71–72.
O15	马高亮. (1996) 按摩治疗中风偏瘫及肩部并发症的体会. 按摩与导引 (3): 14–15.

9

Post-stroke Shoulder Complications: Clinical Evidence for Chinese Medicine Combination Therapies

OVERVIEW

The clinical practice of Chinese medicine often sees several therapy types used in combination, such as Chinese herbal medicine plus acupuncture. An extensive search of nine English and Chinese databases was conducted. After assessment against inclusion criteria, 28 randomised controlled trials which used combinations of Chinese medicine therapies were selected for inclusion. The most common combinations included Chinese herbal medicine with acupuncture therapies. Results showed benefits for the Chinese medicine combination therapies. As meta-analyses were not possible for all different combinations, there is insufficient evidence for various combinations of Chinese medicine therapies.

Introduction

The practice of using two or more Chinese medicine (CM) interventions from different categories together, is common in clinical management of post-stroke complications. Such combined therapies include combinations of two or three CM interventions, e.g. Chinese herbal medicine (CHM), acupuncture, acupressure, electroacupuncture, moxibustion and *tuina* 推拿 therapies. In this chapter, randomised controlled trials (RCTs) of CM combination therapies were identified from literature searches, and were examined to evaluate their efficacy and safety.

Identification of Clinical Studies

A total of 37,141 citations was identified after searching Chinese and English databases. In the end, 30 articles referring to 28 RCTs (C1–C30) that evaluated the combination of two or more CM therapies for post-stroke shoulder complications were included, according to the inclusion criteria (Fig. 9.1). There are four articles which partially reported data from two studies (C1 and C2 were from the same study; C3 and C4 were from the same study); these articles were merged as two studies for analysis.

All RCTs were conducted in China. A total of 2,484 participants was enrolled in these trials. Of the studies that reported participants' gender, there were 1,458 males and 954 female participants. The age of participants ranged from 50 to 80 years (C5), and the median age was 60.5 years.

Of the 28 RCTs, nine studies ([C3 and C4], C6–C13) investigated CM therapies for post-stroke shoulder pain; the remaining 19 RCTs focused on shoulder-hand syndrome (SHS). A number of CM therapies were researched by these studies; these included oral CHM, topical CHM (fomentation, bath and steaming), acupuncture, electroacupuncture, acupressure, moxibustion, *tuina* 推拿 and cupping therapies (see Table 9.1 for a summary). Eight studies ([C3 and C4], C5, C6, C8, C14–C17) compared the combination of two or more CM therapies to routine rehabilitation; the other 20 RCTs ([C1 and C2], C7, C9–C13, C18–C30) studied the add-on effects of CM therapies to routine rehabilitation.

The duration of treatment ranged from 20 days (C19) to eight weeks (C17). CHM treatment was used by 18 studies, with the CHM formulas for each differing. Frequently used herbs in these studies were *hong hua* 红花 (13 studies), *sang zhi* 桑枝 (11 studies), *shen jin cao* 伸筋草 (eight studies), *chuan xiong* 川芎 (eight studies), *dang gui* 当归 (eight studies), *gui zhi* 桂枝 (eight studies), *bai shao* 白芍 (eight

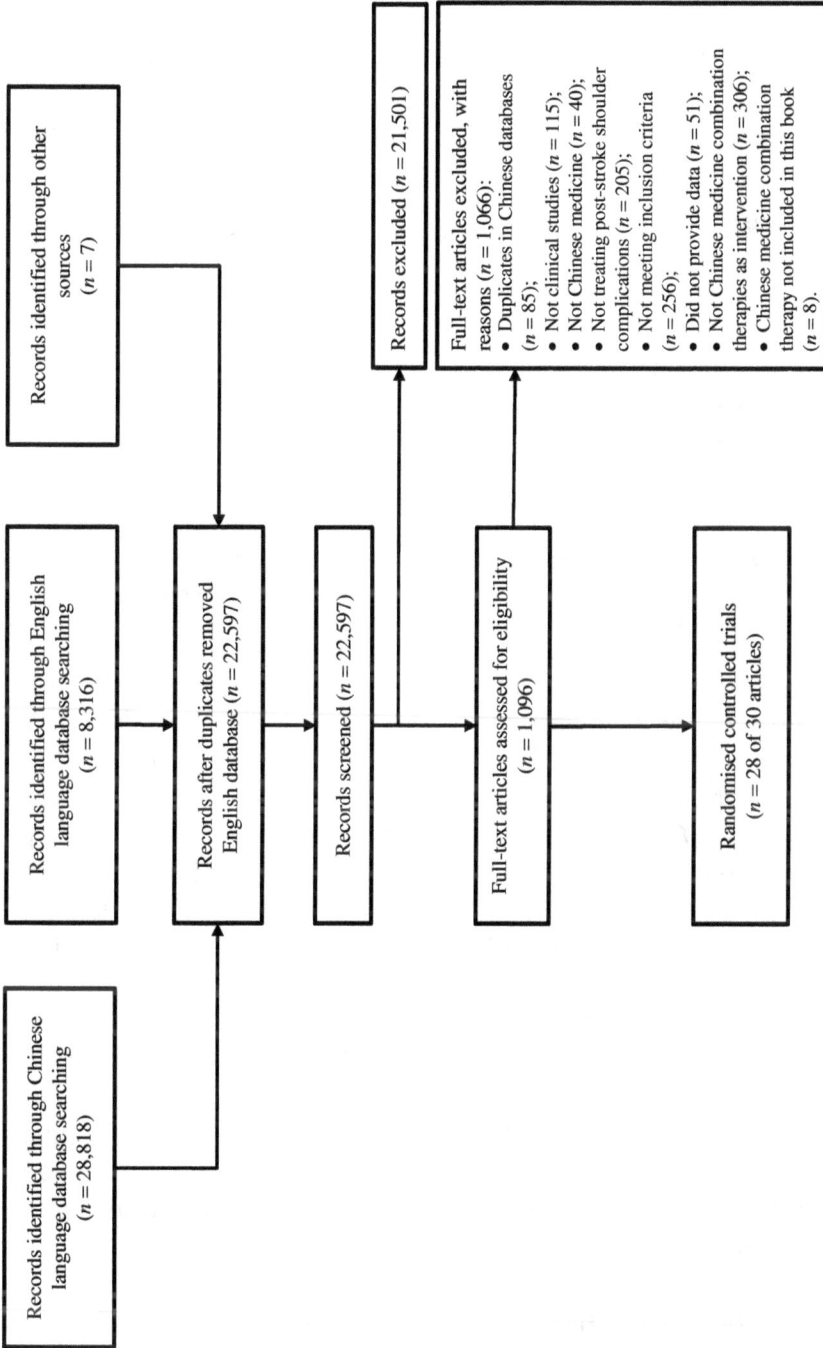

Fig. 9.1 Flowchart of study selection process: Chinese medicine combination therapies.

Records identified through Chinese language database searching (n = 28,818)

Records identified through English language database searching (n = 8,316)

Records identified through other sources (n = 7)

Records after duplicates removed English database (n = 22,597)

Records screened (n = 22,597)

Records excluded (n = 21,501)

Full-text articles assessed for eligibility (n = 1,096)

Full-text articles excluded, with reasons (n = 1,066):
• Duplicates in Chinese databases (n = 85);
• Not clinical studies (n = 115);
• Not Chinese medicine (n = 40);
• Not treating post-stroke shoulder complications (n = 205);
• Not meeting inclusion criteria (n = 256);
• Did not provide data (n = 51);
• Not Chinese medicine combination therapies as intervention (n = 306);
• Chinese medicine combination therapy not included in this book (n = 8).

Randomised controlled trials (n = 28 of 30 articles)

Table 9.1 Summary of Chinese Medicine Combination Therapies

Combination Therapies	No. of Studies	Included Studies
CHM + acupuncture (including electroacupuncture)	10	C18, C20, C5, C22, C7, C23, C15, C24, C11, C26,
CHM + acupressure	3	C19, C12, C30
CHM + acupuncture + *tuina* 推拿 therapy	3	C25, C1, C2 and C29
CHM + *tuina* 推拿 therapy	2	C28, C17
Acupuncture (including electroacupuncture) + *tuina* 推拿 therapy	7	C6, C21, C8, C9, C10, C14, C27
Acupuncture + *tuina* 推拿 therapy + cupping therapy	1	C3 and C4
Moxibustion + tuina 推拿 therapy	1	C16

Note: Two articles (C1 and C2) reported results from one RCT, and another two articles (C3 and C4) reported results from one RCT. Abbreviations: CHM, Chinese herbal medicine; RCT, randomised controlled trial.

studies), *huang qi* 黄芪 (eight studies), *di long* 地龙 (seven studies), *dan shen* 丹参 (six studies), *tao ren* 桃仁 (six studies), *chi shao* 赤芍 (six studies), *tou gu cao* 透骨草 (six studies) and *gan cao* 甘草 (six studies). For the studies which applied acupuncture therapies, there were a total of 48 acupuncture points used, and the most frequently reported points were LI15 *Jianyu* 肩髃 (19 studies), LI11 *Quchi* 曲池 (16 studies), LI4 *Hegu* 合谷 (14 studies), SI9 *Jianzhen* 肩贞 (13 studies), TE14 *Jianliao* 肩髎 (12 studies), TE5 *Waiguan* 外关 (12 studies), LI10 *Shousanli* 手三里 (eight studies), PC6 *Neiguan* 内关 (six studies), GB21 *Jianjing* 肩井 (six studies), TE3 *Zhongzhu* 中渚 (five studies) and LU5 *Chize* 尺泽 (five studies). *Tuina* 推拿 therapy was included in 12 studies; it was applied to the muscles or acupuncture points around the dysfunctional shoulder joint, arm or hand. Cupping therapy (two studies) and moxibustion (one study) were also applied to the local area. See Table 9.1 for a summary of the CM therapies used by all included studies.

Eight studies were identified utilising interventions not commonly practised outside of China; they will not be presented in this chapter.

Risk of Bias Assessment of Included Randomised Controlled Trials

Eight RCTs reported correct randomisation methods, therefore they were assessed as 'low' risk for randomisation sequence generation; one was rated 'high' risk as it used incorrect randomisation methods; and the remaining 19 RCTs were rated 'unclear' risk due to lack of information. Blinding of participants and personnel were judged as 'high' risk of bias for all studies as they were all designed to compare CM therapies to routine rehabilitation therapies without blinding. Blinding of outcome assessors were all rated 'unclear' risk due to lack of information. Incomplete outcome data was assessed as 'low' risk of bias for all studies. For the selective outcome reporting, 25 studies were assessed as 'unclear' risk of bias because these studies reported correct outcomes, as stated in their methodology section, but no protocol could be identified. Another three studies did not state the outcome measures in their methodology section and therefore were rated 'high' risk of bias for this domain. Overall the methodological quality was 'low', thus results should be interpreted with caution. See Table 9.2 for a summary.

Shoulder Subluxation

There was no RCT evaluating the combination of CM therapies with a focus on shoulder subluxation.

Table 9.2   Risk of Bias of Randomised Controlled Trials

Risk of Bias Domain	Low Risk *n* (%)	Unclear Risk *n* (%)	High Risk *n* (%)
Sequence generation	8 (28.6)	19 (67.9)	1 (3.6)
Allocation concealment	2 (7.1)	26 (92.9)	0
Blinding of participants	0	0	28 (100)
Blinding of personnel	0	0	28 (100)
Blinding of outcome assessors	0	28 (100)	0
Incomplete outcome data	28 (100)	0	0
Selective outcome reporting	0	25 (82.3)	3 (10.7)

Shoulder Pain

Nine RCTs ([C3 and C4], C6–C13) were identified from the search which evaluated treatment effects on post-stroke shoulder pain. Among them, three studies ([C3 and C4]. C6, C8) compared CM combined therapies (acupuncture plus *tuina* 推拿, or acupuncture plus *tuina* 推拿 plus cupping) to routine rehabilitation, and six studies (C7, C9–C13) evaluated the add-on effects of CM combined therapies (CHM plus acupuncture or acupressure, or acupuncture plus *tuina* 推拿) to routine rehabilitation. Treatment effects are presented below for each type of therapy.

Acupuncture Plus Tuina 推拿

Electroacupuncture plus *tuina* 推拿 therapies vs.
routine rehabilitation

Two studies (C6, C8) evaluated the combination of electroacupuncture and *tuina* 推拿 therapies, using routine rehabilitation as a comparator, for post-stroke shoulder pain. Treatment was applied for one session each day for a total duration of six weeks and 30 days, respectively. The electroacupuncture and *tuina* 推拿 therapies were conducted on local acupuncture points and muscles. Results of treatment effects are presented below.

Meta-analysis of two studies (C6, C8) showed that the combination of electroacupuncture and *tuina* 推拿 therapies was not different to routine rehabilitation for the outcome of Fugl-Meyer Assessment (FMA) at the end of the treatment phase (MD: 5.36 [−2.84, 13.56], $I^2 = 86\%$).

One study (C8) reported data on the pain visual analogue scale (VAS) of 100 points. When the data was converted to 10 points, it was found that the combination of electroacupuncture and *tuina* 推拿 therapies was superior to routine rehabilitation for pain symptoms (MD: −0.83 [−1.38, −0.28]).

Acupuncture, *tuina* 推拿 therapies and routine
rehabilitation vs. rehabilitation alone

Two RCTs (C9, C10) compared the combination of acupuncture, *tuina* 推拿 therapies and routine rehabilitation to rehabilitation alone. Using FMA as the outcome measure, adding acupuncture and *tuina* 推拿 therapies to routine rehabilitation increased the treatment effects of routine rehabilitation (MD: 6.76 [1.31, 12.21], $I^2 = 82\%$). One study (C10) also reported data on pain VAS; it was found that the combination of acupuncture, *tuina* 推拿 therapy and rehabilitation is more effective for relieving pain compared to routine rehabilitation alone (MD: −1.10 [−1.85, −0.35]).

Acupuncture Plus Tuina 推拿 Plus Cupping Therapies

One study ([C3 and C4]) compared the combination of acupuncture, *tuina* 推拿 and cupping therapies to routine rehabilitation. In addition to acupuncture and *tuina* 推拿 therapies, this study also applied cupping therapy on painful muscle areas. Treatment was conducted once a day for four weeks. Results of this study showed that a combination of acupuncture, *tuina* 推拿 and cupping therapies was more effective than rehabilitation alone for pain VAS (MD: −2.15 [−2.56, −1.74]) and activities of daily living (ADL) using Modified Barthel Index (MBI) (MD: 42.61 [35.63, 49.59]). In this study, the *tuina* 推拿 and cupping therapies were applied mainly focusing on the local shoulder area, while the acupuncture was applied on points located in other areas including GV26 *Renzhong* 人中, PC6 *Neiguan* 内关, HT5 *Tongli* 通里, ST36 *Zusanli* 足三里, GB39 *Xuanzhong* 悬钟, SP6 *Sanyinjiao* 三阴交, KI1 *Yongquan* 涌泉 and HT1 *Jiquan* 极泉.

Chinese Herbal Medicine Plus Acupuncture or Acupressure

Four studies (C7, C11–C13) evaluated the effects of adding CHM and acupuncture or acupressure to routine rehabilitation, in comparison with routine rehabilitation alone. Two of these trials were of oral CHM plus acupuncture (C7, C13), one study investigated the combination of oral CHM and electroacupuncture (C11), and the other study combined topical CHM and acupressure (C12).

Overall meta-analysis showed that using the combination of CHM, acupuncture therapies and routine rehabilitation was more effective than rehabilitation alone for FMA (MD: 4.76 [3.14, 6.39],

$I^2 = 0\%$) (C7, C12) and VAS (MD: −1.67 [−2.18, −1.16], $I^2 = 66\%$) (C7, C11, C13). When using pain (VAS) as the outcome measure, subgroup analysis also confirmed that adding oral CHM and acupuncture to routine rehabilitation is more beneficial than routine rehabilitation alone (MD: −1.77 [−2.43, −1.10], $I^2 = 78\%$) (C7, C13).

A single study (C12) including 120 participants investigated integrating topical CHM fomentation and acupressure on the shoulder area to routine rehabilitation. The results of this study showed benefits of the integrative treatment approach, in terms of both FMA (MD: 5.53 [1.44, 9.62]) and ADL (MBI) (MD: 3.93 [0.92, 6.94]).

In brief, applying CM combination therapies (including acupuncture, CHM, *tuina* 推拿 and cupping therapies) is beneficial for the treatment of post-stroke shoulder pain. In most cases, the CM combination therapies may be as effective as, or even more effective than, routine rehabilitation for certain outcomes. Furthermore, it was confirmed by meta-analyses that adding CM combination therapies to routine rehabilitation increased the treatment effects of routine rehabilitation, in particular for upper limb function and pain symptoms. However, the variation in combinations and small number of included studies requires further investigation in order to achieve conclusive results.

Shoulder-hand Syndrome

In total, 19 studies from 20 publications (C1 and C2 are from the same study) evaluated the effects of CM combination therapies for the treatment of SHS. Among them, five studies (C5, C14–C17) compared CM combination therapies to routine rehabilitation alone, whilst the other 14 studies ([C1 and C2], C18–C30) evaluated the add-on effects of CM combination therapies to routine rehabilitation.

Treatment effects for each type of CM combination therapy are presented below and the results of meta-analyses are summarised in Table 9.3.

Table 9.3 Meta-analysis Results of Chinese Medicine Combination Therapies for Shoulder-hand Syndrome: Chinese Medicine Combination Therapies Plus Routine Rehabilitation vs. Routine Rehabilitation Alone

Chinese Medicine Combined Therapies	Outcomes	No. of Studies	Effects (MD [95% CI])	I2 (%)	No. of Participants	Studies
CHM + acupuncture	FMA	4	10.91 [8.54, 13.28]*	0	354	C18, C24, C22, C23
	VAS	2	−4.12 [−5.23, −3.01]*	91	182	C18, C26
CHM + acupressure	FMA	2	6.36 [3.50, 9.22]*	0	136	C19, C30
	VAS	2	−1.35 [−2.24, −0.47]*	68	136	C19, C30
CHM + acupuncture + tuina 推拿	FMA	2	7.13 [6.02, 8.23]*	0	187	C25, (C1 and C2)

*Statistically significant. Abbreviations: CHM, Chinese herbal medicine; CI, confidence interval; FMA, Fugl-Meyer Assessment; MD, mean difference; VAS, visual analogue scale.

Chinese Herbal Medicine Plus Acupuncture

Two RCTs compared the combination of CHM and acupuncture to routine rehabilitation. One of these studies (C15) used oral CHM, and the other one (C5) used topical CHM (bath). Results from the oral CHM plus acupuncture study (C15) showed the combination of oral CHM and acupuncture was more effective than routine rehabilitation for upper limb FMA (MD: 10.50 [7.19, 13.81]), VAS (MD: −1.20 [−1.92, −0.48]) and ADL (MD: 15.70 [12.36, 19.04]). The study of topical CHM only reported effective rate data, but without clear criteria of assessing the effective rate (C5).

Six RCTs investigated integrating CHM, acupuncture and routine rehabilitation, compared to routine rehabilitation alone. Of these, three studies (C18, C20, C24) were of oral CHM and acupuncture, two studies (C22, C23) evaluated topical CHM steam therapy plus acupuncture, and another one (C26) assessed the combination of oral CHM, topical CHM and acupuncture. Meta-analysis showed the integrative treatment was more effective than routine rehabilitation alone for upper limb FMA (MD: 10.91 [8.54, 13.28], I^2 = 0%) (C18, C22–C24), and VAS (MD: –4.12 [–5.23, –3.01], I2 = 91%) (C18, C26). In addition, data on ADL (MBI) was reported by one study (C22), and the result was also in favour of integrative medicine treatment (MD: 7.75 [3.82, 11.68]).

Chinese Herbal Medicine Plus Acupressure

Two RCTs (C19, C30) investigated the combination of CHM and acupressure, integrated with routine rehabilitation, compared to rehabilitation alone. Both studies reported data on FMA and pain VAS. Meta-analysis results showed that adding CHM and acupressure to routine rehabilitation could significantly increase the effects of rehabilitation, in terms of upper limb FMA (MD: 6.36 [3.50, 9.22], I^2 = 0%) (C19, C30) and VAS (MD: –1.35 [–2.24, –0.47], I^2 = 68%) (C19, C30).

Chinese Herbal Medicine Plus Tuina 推拿

Comparing the combination of CHM and *tuina* 推拿 therapy to rehabilitation, one study (C17) reported data on upper limb FMA. It was found that the combination of CHM and *tuina* 推拿 therapy was more effective than rehabilitation alone (MD: 8.86 [6.34, 11.38]).

One RCT (C28) evaluated integrating CHM and *tuina* 推拿 therapy with rehabilitation, using rehabilitation alone as the comparator. This study reported data on upper limb FMA and VAS. It found that the integration of therapies was superior to rehabilitation for both outcomes: FMA (MD: 5.84 [3.07, 8.61]) and VAS (MD: –1.50 [–1.92, –1.08]).

Chinese Herbal Medicine Plus Acupuncture Plus Tuina 推拿

When combining CHM, acupuncture and *tuina* 推拿 therapy, three RCTs ([C1 and C2], C25, C29) integrated these three therapies with rehabilitation and compared it to rehabilitation alone. All three studies used topical CHM treatment including CHM steaming and CHM bath.

Two studies ([C1 and C2], C25) reported data on upper limb FMA; a meta-analysis showed integrative therapy was more effective than rehabilitation alone (MD: 7.13 [6.02, 8.23], I^2 = 0%). Visual analogue scale was reported by one study (C25), and shoulder joint range of motion (ROM) was reported by another study ([C1 and C2]). Results of these outcomes were also in favour of the integrative medicine: VAS (MD: −0.80 [−1.36, −0.24]) (C25) and ROM (MD: −0.52 [−0.68, −0.36]) ([C1 and C2]).

Acupuncture Plus Tuina 推拿

Two studies (C21, C27) evaluated integrating acupuncture, *tuina* 推拿 therapy and rehabilitation compared to rehabilitation alone. Meta-analysis was not possible. Single-study results showed that the integrative medicine treatment was more effective than rehabilitation alone for FMA (MD: 22.70 [18.02, 27.38]) (C27), pain VAS (MD: −3.28 [−4.05, −2.51]) (C21) and shoulder ROM (MD: −0.65 [−1.03, −0.27]) (C27).

Electroacupuncture Plus Tuina 推拿

One study (C14) compared the combination of electroacupuncture and *tuina* 推拿 therapy to rehabilitation alone. Results showed the combination of CM therapy was more effective than rehabilitation alone in terms of upper limb FMA (MD: 16.01 [14.69, 17.33]) and VAS (MD: −2.11 [−2.82, −1.40]).

Moxibustion Plus Tuina 推拿

One study (C16) compared the combination of moxibustion and *tuina* 推拿 therapy to rehabilitation alone. Results showed the combination of CM therapy was more effective than rehabilitation alone in terms of upper limb FMA (MD: 10.10 [9.11, 11.09]), VAS (MD: −1.29 [−1.61, −0.97]) and ADL (MD: 11.97 [7.57, 16.37]).

In summary, applying a combination of different CM therapies (e.g. acupuncture, acupressure, electroacupuncture, CHM, *tuina* 推拿 and moxibustion) is beneficial for the treatment of post-stroke SHS. Based on single-study results, combined CM treatment is more effective than routine rehabilitation alone; however, no meta-analyses could be conducted. On the other hand, meta-analysis confirmed integrating CM combination therapy to routine rehabilitation increases the treatment effects of routine rehabilitation alone, in terms of upper limb function (assessed by FMA) and pain symptoms (assessed by VAS).

Safety of Chinese Medicine Combined Therapy

Of all the included RCTs, three studies ([C1 and C2], C13, C29) mentioned adverse event information. Two of them ([C1 and C2], C29) evaluated the combination of topical CHM, acupuncture and *tuina* 推拿, and one (C13) investigated oral CHM plus acupuncture. All three studies reported no occurrence of adverse events during the trial and thus concluded that CM combination therapies were safe for the management of post-stroke shoulder complications.

Evidence for Chinese Medicine Combination Therapies Commonly Used in Clinical Practice

Many RCTs have evaluated combinations of CM therapies for post-stroke shoulder complications, focusing on shoulder pain and SHS. The effects of CM combination therapies for shoulder subluxation have not been evaluated by clinical studies.

Although any combination of CM therapies has not been particularly recommended by clinical guidelines (see Chapter 2 for a summary), our review of clinical RCTs found that two or more different CM therapies, including acupuncture (or electroacupuncture), *tuina* 推拿 therapy, CHM (oral or topical) or moxibustion, had been combined together as management for shoulder pain and SHS.

Summary of Clinical Evidence for Chinese Medicine Combination Therapies

This section evaluated the combination of two or more CM therapies used in post-stroke shoulder complication management. Among all included studies, CHM plus acupuncture is the most commonly used combination, followed by the combination of acupuncture and *tuina* 推拿 therapy. CHM was administered as oral and all forms of topical methods (bath, steam, fomentation and topical application). Acupuncture therapy (including electroacupuncture and acupressure) is the most commonly used therapy; it was included in 85% of the assessed studies (24 of 28). Of the studies investigating the combination of CHM and other therapies, most did not provide formula names. The herb ingredients of their formulas are consistent with those frequently used in those studies which only evaluated CHM (see Chapter 5). The most frequently used herbs are *hong hua* 红花, *sang zhi* 桑枝, *shen jin cao* 伸筋草, *chuan xiong* 川芎, *dang gui* 当归, *gui zhi* 桂枝, *bai shao* 白芍, *huang qi* 黄芪, *di long* 地龙, *dan shen* 丹参, *tao ren* 桃仁, *chi shao* 赤芍, *tou gu cao* 透骨草 and *gan cao* 甘草. Further, acupuncture therapies of included studies were conducted focusing on the local points of the shoulder area and upper limb, including LI15 *Jianyu* 肩髃, SI9 *Jianzhen* 肩贞, TE14 *Jianliao* 肩髎, GB21 *Jianjing* 肩井, LI11 *Quchi* 曲池, LI10 *Shousanli* 手三里, LU5 *Chize* 尺泽, TE5 *Waiguan* 外关, PC6 *Neiguan* 内关 and LI4 *Hegu* 合谷. *Tuina* 推拿therapy was also consistent with the methods introduced in Chapter 8; it was often applied to the muscles or acupuncture points around the dysfunctional shoulder joint, arm or hand. Syndrome differentiation was not essential for these studies. The treatment duration varied from one week to eight weeks, with four weeks being the most common duration.

For the management of shoulder pain, there was evidence from meta-analyses supporting the add-on effects for upper limb function (FMA) of acupuncture plus *tuina* 推拿 therapies and CHM plus acupuncture/acupressure therapies, as well as the add-on effects for shoulder joint pain severity (VAS) of CHM plus acupuncture therapies. In terms of patients' activities of daily living (ADL), there was evidence from single studies supporting the add-on effects of CM combination therapy including acupuncture plus *tuina* 推拿 plus cupping therapies, and CHM fomentation plus acupressure therapies.

Similarly, for the management of SHS, there was evidence from meta-analyses supporting the add-on effects for upper limb function (FMA) of CHM plus acupuncture therapies, CHM plus acupressure therapies, and CHM, plus acupuncture, plus *tuina* 推拿 therapies, as well as the add-on effects for shoulder joint pain severity (VAS) of CHM plus acupressure therapies. The benefit of adding CM combination therapy to routine rehabilitation for shoulder joint movement (ROM) was only supported by single studies, including the combination of acupuncture and *tuina* 推拿 therapies, and CHM, plus acupuncture, plus *tuina* 推拿 therapies.

Few of the included studies compared combinations of CM interventions with routine rehabilitation. There was no meta-analysis evidence showing superior effects of CM combination therapy.

Our review of clinical studies did not include the studies comparing two or more CM therapies to one CM therapy (e.g. CHM plus acupuncture vs. acupuncture); therefore, it is unclear whether adding multiple CM therapies is more beneficial than only adding one of them to routine rehabilitation.

Chinese medicine combination therapies seem safe for the management of post-stroke shoulder complications. Based on the evidence of individual CM therapies (see Chapters 5, 7 and 8) and the evidence of combination therapies, practitioners could consider incorporating them into clinical practice.

References to Included Clinical Studies

Study No.	References
C1	李乐军, 陈丽萍, 刘晓丽, 肖辉, 黄蓉, 常辉, 宋雅琼, 乔本玉, 李玉梅. (2013) 中药泡洗结合针灸推拿和康复训练对脑梗塞后肩手综合征患者的生活质量影响. 时珍国医国药 (1): 173–175.

(Continued)

(Continued)

Study No.	References
C2	李乐军, 陈丽萍, 刘晓丽, 肖辉, 黄蓉, 常辉, 宋雅琼, 乔本玉. (2012) 中药泡洗结合针灸推拿和康复训练治疗脑梗死后肩手综合征的临床研究. 辽宁中医杂志 (10): 1935–1937.
C3	黄锦军, 粟胜勇, 雷龙鸣, 胡玉英, 邓柏颖, 苏赐明, 甘业进, 戴李国, 吴舸. (2009) 推拿、针刺、拔火罐治疗中风偏瘫后肩痛及对全血黏度的影响. 陕西中医 (5): 591–593.
C4	黄锦军, 粟胜勇, 雷龙鸣, 胡玉英, 邓柏颖, 苏赐明, 甘业进, 戴李国, 吴舸. (2009) 中医综合疗法治疗中风偏瘫致肩痛及上肢活动障碍的临床研究. 广西中医药 (2): 28–30.
C5	和亚群, 黄桂英. (2015) 脑卒中后肩手综合征采用针刺结合中药泡洗治疗的临床效果. 中国医学工程 (1): 163.
C6	李宁, 田丰玮, 王成伟, 喻鹏铭, 周熙, 文谦, 乔秀兰, 黄露. (2012) 电针配合推拿治疗脑卒中后肩痛:双中心随机对照试验. 中国针灸 (2): 101–105.
C7	端木香凤. (2015) 针刺联合身痛逐瘀汤治疗中风偏瘫后肩痛临床研究. 河南中医 (1): 67–69.
C8	刘悦, 凌方明, 龙目恒. (2002) 针刺推拿治疗偏瘫肩痛疗效体会. 中国临床康复 (18): 2742–2743.
C9	温元强, 陈立, 温伯平. (2011) 针灸推拿联合康复疗法治疗脑卒中后肩痛疗效评价. 中国中医药信息杂志 (9): 67–68.
C10	李志宇. (2014) 针灸推拿联合康复疗法治疗脑卒中后肩痛疗效探究. 中国伤残医学 (22): 162–163.
C11	钱仁义. (2008) 中西医结合治疗卒中后肩痛临床观察. 中国实用神经疾病杂志 (7): 131–132.
C12	洪敏巧, 沈雪琴, 元国芬. (2012) 中药热敷联合穴位按压治疗脑卒中后肩痛的效果观察. 护理与康复 (6): 568–570.
C13	倪烨, 陆俊, 肖晓, 张汉新. (2012) 自拟活血祛痰通络汤治疗中风恢复期偏瘫肩痛38例. 四川中医 (10): 101–102.
C14	刘爱国, 吴秀玲. (2009) 针灸推拿治疗脑卒中后肩手综合征63例疗效观察. 河北中医 (2): 262–263.
C15	于振章, 侯瀚翔. (2012) 针药结合治疗脑卒中后肩手综合征临床观察. 中国民间疗法 (10): 53–54.
C16	余智. (2014) 推拿结合循经往返灸治疗脑卒中后肩手综合征临床研究. 中医学报 (11): 1689–1691.

(Continued)

(Continued)

Study No.	References
C17	蔡智瑛. (2014) 穴位按摩结合药熨治疗脑卒中后肩—手综合征的中医护理分析. 按摩与康复医学 (2): 126–127.
C18	廉全荣, 封臻. (2014) 补气化痰通络法结合针刺治疗脑卒中后肩手综合征57例. 陕西中医 (2): 146–147.
C19	郝重耀, 杨发明. (2013) 磁圆梅针联合中药熏蒸治疗肩手综合征疗效观察. 中国中医药信息杂志 (12): 69–70.
C20	毛光兰, 贾奎. (2015) 加味补阳还五汤联合针刺养老穴治疗脑卒中后肩-手综合征疗效观察. 新乡医学院学报 (1): 62–64.
C21	钱雪峰. (2011) 在肩手综合症康复治疗中运用针灸推拿的疗效观察. 按摩与康复医学 (30): 62.
C22	任扬, 赵义纯. (2013) 针刺结合中药熏洗治疗脑卒中后肩-手综合征疗效观察. 内蒙古中医药 (14): 42–43.
C23	吕红姣, 崔丽笙. (2013) 针刺联合中药熏蒸治疗脑卒中后肩手综合征的效果观察. 护理与康复 (7): 696–698.
C24	张方, 李文杰. (2009) 针药结合治疗中风后肩手综合征60例. 中国中医急症 (6): 974–975.
C25	彭慧渊, 王寅, 王本国, 徐帮杰, 赵明华, 杨楠. (2014) 中风后肩痛中医诊疗方案治疗肩手综合征Ⅰ期疗效观察. 现代中西医结合杂志 (7): 687–689.
C26	贾爱明, 艾群, 刘耘, 刁凤声, 毕伟莲, 董玉宽. (2013) 中药联合针刺治疗脑卒中后肩手综合征的疗效观察. 大连医科大学学报 (3): 264–267.
C27	顾力华, 石丽琼, 陈奇刚, 陈红波, 周建英. (2014) 中医综合治疗对脑卒中后肩手综合征Ⅰ期患者肩关节功能的影响. 中国伤残医学 (19): 155–156.
C28	刘路明, 包译. (2012) 传统康复方法分期治疗肩手综合征 50 例. 云南中医中药杂志 (9): 43–44.
C29	谭绍超. (2011) 缺血性中风恢复早期肩手综合征综合治疗临床研究. [Thesis]. 长春中医药大学..
C30	于川, 陈东霞, 孙静波. (2013) 自拟药棒穴位疗法结合康复训练治疗脑卒中后 1 期肩手综合征 25 例. 中医外治杂志 (5): 42621.

10

Summary of Evidence

OVERVIEW

Chinese medicine therapies have been used to treat stroke and its complications for a long time, although post-stroke shoulder complications, including shoulder pain, subluxation and shoulder-hand syndrome, have not been treated as independent conditions in ancient China. In the recent decades, a significant number of clinical studies have been conducted to evaluate Chinese medicine therapies. Findings from clinical evidence revealed promising benefits of oral and topical Chinese herbal medicine, acupuncture therapies and other Chinese medicine therapies. This chapter provides a 'whole evidence' analysis in investigating Chinese medicine for the management of post-stroke shoulder complications. The limitations of the available evidence are discussed and future directions are identified for clinical and experimental research.

Introduction

Stroke is currently the leading cause of neurological disability in adults. It can result in high levels of residual disability that can persist for months, years or the remainder of the individual's life. Effective rehabilitation interventions initiated early after stroke can enhance the recovery process and minimise functional disability. Post-stroke shoulder complications (shoulder pain, shoulder subluxation and shoulder-hand syndrome (SHS)) have been increasingly researched since they may negatively affect rehabilitation outcomes.

Shoulder subluxation is a common occurrence after stroke and can be due to muscle weakness or spasticity. Post-stroke pain is related to multiple factors, including central and peripheral mechanisms, psychological factors and autonomic input. Post-stroke SHS has been determined as complex regional pain syndrome (CRPS) type I, which is prevalent in hemiplegic patients. Prevention is the most important management of post-stroke shoulder subluxation and pain. Once the full pain syndrome has developed, treatment should commence. Chinese medicine (CM) therapies play a role to assist conventional therapies in the management of post-stroke shoulder complications.

In order to provide a 'whole evidence' evaluation, in this book we analysed the evidence of CM therapies from all type of literature for the three main post-stroke shoulder complications: shoulder pain, shoulder subluxation and SHS.

A review of clinical guidelines and textbooks identified a range of CM treatments that have been recommended, or suggested, including oral and topical Chinese herbal medicine (CHM), acupuncture and traditional Chinese *tuina* 推拿 therapy (Chapter 2).

Considering post-stroke shoulder complications have not been specifically discussed in history, to identify the CM treatment in classical literature is challenging. Therefore, we searched classical literature from an angle of overall stroke and post-stroke motor function impairment (Chapter 3). Numerous clinical trials of CM therapies have been conducted in China. Some of these studies have shown promising results. Using a systematic review approach, clinical evidence has been found to support the use of CHM (Chapter 5), acupuncture-related therapies (Chapter 7), *tuina* 推拿 therapy and cupping therapy (Chapter 8), and some combination of multiple CM therapies (Chapter 9). The herbs that were used most frequently in the randomised controlled trials (RCTs) have shown actions in experimental studies, which shed light on their probable mechanisms of action (Chapter 6).

Chinese Medicine Syndrome Differentiation

Clarified CM syndrome differentiation of post-stroke shoulder complications is seldom seen in the present clinical guidelines or textbooks.

The commonly applied syndrome differentiation in clinical practice is that of meridian stroke 中经络, including Wind-Fire uprising, Wind-Phlegm obstructing the collaterals, Phlegm-Heat heat and excess in the *fu* 腑 organ, *qi* 气 deficiency with Blood stasis and *yin* 阴 deficiency with Wind.

Syndrome differentiation was rarely reported by the clinical studies. Only a few studies utilising oral CHM considered selecting CHM formulas/herbs according to syndrome differentiation (Chapter 5). Of them, Blood stasis and Phlegm stagnation were the most commonly reported syndromes. Although some clinical studies may have used syndrome differentiation for treatment selection (especially if multiple formulas were used in the study), results are usually reported in aggregate and not by syndrome. Therefore, it is not possible to establish efficacy of treatments according to syndrome types.

Among the studies of acupuncture-related therapies (Chapter 7) and other CM therapies (Chapter 8), syndrome differentiation was not reported by the included studies. It is unclear whether the principle of selecting acupuncture points according to syndrome was applied in these studies.

Chinese Herbal Medicine

This section summarises the evidence from Chapters 2, 3, 5 and 9.

Chinese herbal medicine therapies have been suggested by all forms of evidence in the treatment of post-stroke shoulder complications. Both oral and topical CHM therapies have been recommended by contemporary textbooks and guidelines, and also evaluated in clinical studies. Oral CHM has been recorded in classical literature as the treatment for stroke and its motor function impairment, e.g. one formula (*Shi wei cuo san* 十味锉散) was stated as treating Blood deficiency type *zhong feng* 中风 upper limb pain and difficult movement (治中风血弱, 臂痛连及筋骨, 举动艰难). However, our search of *Zhong Hua Yi Dian* 中华医典 version 5 did not identify any citations with topical CHM.

The CM aetiology of *zhong feng* 中风 has been changed from external Wind attack in combination with *qi* 气 deficiency to internal factors, in particular Liver *yang* upraising 肝阳上亢. This internal factors' causality is similar to that defined in current clinical practice. In accordance with the historical development of our understanding of disease, CHM treatment principles also switched from eliminating external Wind to dealing with internal factors. In addition, post-stroke shoulder complications were not treated as a certain disease in history, and pain management was not a priority in the *zhong feng* 中风 treatment. As a result, the formulas commonly used in classical literature are not completely consistent with what are in use at present. In terms of the most frequently used herbs, it noted that some herbs have the function of nourishing Blood and removing Blood stasis, e.g. *dang gui* 当归, *chuan xiong* 川芎, *di huang* 地黄 and *niu xi* 牛膝; some herbs can tonify *qi* 气, *yang* 阳 or Spleen, e.g. *fu zi* 附子, *rou gui* 肉桂, *ren shen* 人参, *bai zhu* 白术, *fu ling* 茯苓, *bai fu ling* 白茯苓, *huang qi* 黄芪 and ginger 生姜; some herbs can reduce Phlegm, e.g. *ban xia* 半夏, *tian nan xing/dan nan xing/nan xing* 天南星/胆南星/南星 and *zhu li* 竹沥; some herbs may eliminate Wind, e.g. *fang feng* 防风, *qiang huo* 羌活, *ma huang* 麻黄 and *qin jiu* 秦艽; and some herbs could work for unblocking meridians, e.g. *tian ma* 天麻 (see Tables 3.5 and 3.6 for more information).

In the evaluation of modern literature evidence of CHM for post-stroke shoulder complications, SHS has been the most investigated by clinical trials of CHM. The analysis of the clinical studies found variation in formulas and routes of administration of CHM, and diversity in the outcomes reported. Topical CHM was the most frequently investigated CHM; it was used in the form of CHM bath therapy, CHM fomentation, CHM steam therapy and CHM external application in clinical studies. In terms of the treatment effects, some promising clinical evidence was seen with oral CHM, topical CHM and the combination of oral and topical CHM for all the three types of post-stroke shoulder complications. It is noted that topical CHM may play the most important role in the management of post-stroke shoulder complications. Details are presented in Chapter 5. In addition, the herbs used both orally and topically that may have contributed to the positive effects seen include *chuan xiong* 川芎, *hong hua* 红花, *dang gui* 当归, *chi shao* 赤芍, *ji xue teng* 鸡血藤

and *sang zhi* 桑枝 (see Table 5.12 for more information). Some herbs are more often used topically, which may have contributed to the positive effects; these are *shen jin cao* 伸筋草, *tou gu cao* 透骨草, *ai ye* 艾叶, *mo yao* 没药 and *ru xiang* 乳香 (see Tables 5.7 and 5.18 for more information). Practitioners may consider these herbs when preparing prescriptions for patients with post-stroke shoulder complications. Few side effects were reported with CHM and therefore it seems safe; however, it was noted that most of the included studies did not mention information of adverse events.

The analysis of treatment effects showed that oral and topical CHM were effective for managing post-stroke shoulder complications; in particular, they were only administered as an effective add-on therapy to conventional rehabilitations and routine care. However, the heterogeneity in the meta-analyses indicates that there was considerable variability in each result. At least part of this variability was due to the use of different CHMs but it was not possible to determine which CHM produced the greatest effect since most studies tested different formulas, even though many were based on similar ingredients. Other factors influencing the interpretation of the results of the clinical studies were the relatively poor reporting of trial design and methods, and the lack of blinding in most studies. Information of adverse events was not reported in many studies. These aspects reduced confidence in the accuracy of the reported results and influenced the downgrading of the quality of the evidence in the Grading of Recommendations Assessment, Development and Evaluation (GRADE) assessments.

Chinese Herbal Medicine Formulas in Key Clinical Guidelines and Textbooks: Classical Literature and Clinical Studies

Table 10.1 summarises the CHM formulas described in clinical guidelines and textbooks (Chapter 2), classical literature (Chapter 3) and clinical studies (Chapter 5). Assessment was based on formula name. It is likely that formulas with the same or similar herb ingredients, but with different formula names, were included. As assessment of similarity of formulas is complex and was not undertaken, the

Table 10.1   Summary of Chinese Herbal Medicine Formulas

Formula Name	Evidence in Clinical Guidelines and Textbooks (Chapter 2)	Evidence in Classical Literature (Chapter 3) (No. of Citations)	Included in Clinical Studies (Chapter 5) (No. of Studies)			Included in Combination Therapies (Chapter 9)
			RCTs	CCTs	Non-controlled Studies	
Oral CHM						
Tian ma gou teng yin 天麻钩藤饮加减	Yes	0	0	0	0	0
Hua tan tong luo tang 化痰通络汤	Yes	0	0	0	0	0
Xing lou cheng qi tang 星蒌承气汤	Yes	0	0	0	0	0
Bu yang huan wu tang 补阳还五汤加减	Yes	0 (2)*	4	0	1	1
Zhen gan xi feng tang 镇肝熄风汤	Yes	0	0	0	0	0
Shi wei cuo san 十味锉散	No	2	0	0	0	0
Shen tong zhu yu tang 身痛逐瘀汤	No	0	2	0	0	1
Huang qi gui zhi wu wu tang 黄芪桂枝五物汤	No	0	2	0	0	0
Topical CHM						
CHM bath therapy: *Fu fang tong luo ye* 复方通络液	Yes	0	0	0	0	0

*Bu yang huan wu tang 补阳还五汤 was identified in classical literature in the citations of 'possibly post-stroke shoulder complications,' since these citations did not specify shoulder symptoms. Abbreviations: CCT, controlled clinical trial; CHM, Chinese herbal medicine; RCT, randomised controlled trial.

actual number of formulas using the same ingredients may be higher than what are listed below.

Based on our analysis, the formulas recorded in classical literature are not completely consistent with those being commonly used in current clinical practice. *Bu yang huan wu tang* 补阳还五汤 is the only formula that had evidence in all types of literature. It is recommended as a key formula for post-stroke motor function impairment in clinical practice, it is shown in classical literature (although not the most frequent one), and it has been proven effective for pain relief in SHS by clinical studies.

Furthermore, topical CHM was used in the majority of clinical studies. However, most of these studies did not provide the name of the formula, so it is difficult for clinicians to replicate the clinical research in their practice. Researchers should take this point into consideration in their future work.

Acupuncture and Related Therapies

This section summarises the evidence from Chapters 2, 3, 7 and 9.

Acupuncture therapies have a long history of use for the clinical management of post-stroke shoulder complications. Acupuncture therapies have been described in both the classical and contemporary literature, and have been researched in clinical studies, with over 130 studies meeting the eligibility criteria.

Consistency was seen across all forms of evidence in terms of the acupuncture therapies used to treat post-stroke shoulder complications. Manual acupuncture and moxibustion are recommended in clinical textbooks and guidelines, have been cited in the classical literature, and were evaluated in clinical research.

Our search of *Zhong Hua Yi Dian* 中华医典 found that the acupuncture and moxibustion treatments for *zhong feng* 中风 date back to the Tang dynasty, and has been continually used until current clinical practice. In ancient China, most of the acupuncture treatments were combined with moxibustion. Three promising acupuncture points for shoulder complications were LI15 *Jianyu* 肩髃, GB21 *Jianjing* 肩井 and LI11 *Quchi* 曲池 (see Table 3.9). In particular, LI15 *Jianyu* 肩髃 could be considered as the key acupuncture point for treating and preventing post-stroke shoulder complications.

In clinical studies, acupuncture has shown promising clinical effects for all shoulder complications, and moxibustion combining acupuncture has proven beneficial for shoulder pain and SHS when they were used as add-on therapies. Other than these two therapies, some modern forms of acupuncture-related therapies including electroacupuncture, scalp acupuncture, floating acupuncture 浮针, wrist-ankle acupuncture 腕踝针 and acupressure have all been evaluated and proven beneficial for shoulder symptoms. The most frequently used acupuncture points for these three complications are LI15 *Jianyu* 肩髃, TE14 *Jianliao* 肩髎 and SI9 *Jianzhen* 肩贞. The commonly recommended acupoints in clinical studies are located in the Large intestine meridian 手阳明大肠经, Small intestine meridian 手太阳小肠经 and Triple energizer meridian 手少阳三焦经. These points are consistent with those that may have contributed to positive effects in the meta-analyses. Practitioners can feel confident that there is a long history of use to support the selection of these points in post-stroke shoulder complications. In addition, few adverse events were reported in the treatment groups, suggesting that acupuncture-related therapies were well tolerated and can be considered a safe treatment option for people with post-stroke shoulder complications.

Similar to the CHM studies, there were inadequacies in the reporting of trial methodology; the studies were not blinded and safety data were inadequately reported. Therefore, the assessment of the quality of the evidence was rated down in the GRADE tables for acupuncture and electroacupuncture.

Acupuncture-related Therapies in Key Clinical Guidelines and Textbooks: Classical Literature and Clinical Studies

Overall, consistency was seen in the interventions cited across all evidence types (see Table 10.2 for a summary). Acupuncture and moxibustion have a long history of use for post-stroke shoulder complications, with both being cited in classical literature. Both interventions have been recommended in clinical guidelines. Over 150 clinical studies have evaluated acupuncture, and 15 have evaluated moxibustion.

More recent developments in acupuncture-related therapies have been investigated in clinical research including electroacupuncture, scalp acupuncture, floating acupuncture and acupressure.

Table 10.2 Summary of Acupuncture-related Therapies

Acupuncture Therapy	Included in Clinical Guidelines and Textbooks (Chapter 2)	Included in Classical Literature (Chapter 3) (No. of Citations)	Included in Clinical Studies (Chapter 7) (No. of Studies)			Included in Combination Therapies (Chapter 9) (No. of Studies)
			RCTs*	CCTs*	Non-controlled Studies*	
Body acupuncture	Yes	11	101	3	31	18
Moxibustion	Yes	8	9	4	1	1

*Some studies used more than one intervention e.g. acupuncture plus moxibustion. These are counted separately in this table. Abbreviations: CCTs, controlled clinical trials; RCTs, randomised controlled trials.

In order to summarise which traditional acupuncture points were used for acupuncture and/or moxibustion treatment, all the points that were recommended in Chapter 2 and the points most frequently used in the randomised controlled trials (RCTs) in Chapter 7 were included in Table 10.3. The use of these points was cross-referenced to other clinical trial types and other chapters.

The points listed for acupuncture in Chapter 2 (LI15 *Jianyu* 肩髃, TE14 *Jianliao* 肩髎, SI9 *Jianzhen* 肩贞, (EX) *Jianqian* 肩前, *Ashi* points 阿是穴, TE2 *Yemen* 液门, TE4 *Yangchi* 阳池 and SI4 *Wangu* 腕骨) were recommended to be used for acupuncture, with moxibustion applied if needed. Among these points, only one point (LI15 *Jianyu* 肩髃) was also suggested in classical literature. On the other hand, some points were often seen in classical literature but not recommended in Chapter 2 (e.g. GB21 *Jianjing* 肩井, LI11 *Quchi* 曲池, LI14 *Binao* 臂臑 and LI10 *Shousanli* 手三里). Clinical research has investigated acupuncture therapies using various points, including all the abovementioned points with the exception of TE2 *Yemen* 液门. According to the summary in Table 10.3, it is noted that the most frequently used points in clinical research are LI15 *Jianyu* 肩髃, LI11 *Quchi* 曲池, LI14 *Binao* 臂臑, LI10 *Shousanli* 手三里, TE14 *Jianliao* 肩髎 and SI9 *Jianzhen* 肩贞. These points are also shown in the list of most frequent acupuncture points used in studies from favourable meta-analyses (see Tables 7.6 and 7.11 for more information);

Table 10.3   Summary of Acupuncture Points Included

Acupuncture Point	Clinical Guidelines and Textbooks (Chapter 2)	Classical Literature (Chapter 3) (No. of Citations)	Clinical Studies in Chapter 7 (No. of Studies)			Combination Therapies (Chapter 9) (No. of Studies)
			RCTs	CCTs	Non-controlled Studies*	
Acupuncture						
LI15 Jianyu 肩髃	Yes	32	53	2	21	18
TE14 Jianliao 肩髎	Yes	0	35	1	12	11
SI9 Jianzhen 肩贞	Yes	0	32	2	10	12
(EX) Jianqian 肩前	Yes	0	12	0	7	4
Ashi points 阿是穴	Yes	0	16	0	3	7
TE2 Yemen 液门	Yes	0	0	0	0	0
TE4 Yangchi 阳池	Yes	0	5	0	1	2
SI4 Wangu 腕骨	Yes	0	2	0	0	0
GB21 Jianjing 肩井	No	10	11	0	6	4
LI11 Quchi 曲池	No	41	44	3	14	15
LI14 Binao 臂臑	No	32	24	2	10	2
LI10 Shousanli 手三里	No	22	24	1	13	8
Moxibustion						
LI15 Jianyu 肩髃	Yes	32	5	0	4	0
TE14 Jianliao 肩髎	Yes	0	4	0	2	0
SI9 Jianzhen 肩贞	Yes	0	4	0	1	0
(EX) Jianqian 肩前	Yes	0	1	0	3	0
Ashi points 阿是穴	Yes	0	4	0	0	0
TE2 Yemen 液门	Yes	0	0	0	0	0
TE4 Yangchi 阳池	Yes	0	1	0	0	0
SI4 Wangu 腕骨	Yes	0	1	0	0	0

*Some studies used more than one intervention e.g. acupuncture plus moxibustion. These are counted separately in this table. Abbreviations: CCTs, controlled clinical trials; RCTs, randomised controlled trials.

therefore they may be considered in clinical practice for managing post-stroke shoulder complications.

Other Chinese Medicine Therapies

Of the range of other CM therapies that may be used to treat post-stroke shoulder complications, *tuina* 推拿 therapy (Chinese massage) has been recommended in contemporary texts and evaluated in clinical evidence, and cupping therapy has been recorded in classical literature and also evaluated in clinical studies. However, no therapy has evidence from all forms of literature. See Table 10.4 for a summary.

Tuina 推拿 therapy, when used as an add-on therapy to routine rehabilitation, has been found beneficial for upper limb function, shoulder joint range of motion (ROM) (lifting) and pain symptoms of shoulder subluxation and pain. For SHS, the current evidence shows that adding *tuina* 推拿 therapy to routine rehabilitation could improve patients' daily activity; however, there is insufficient evidence supporting its use for relieving pain and improving upper limb function. *Tuina* 推拿 therapy is usually applied on the local shoulder muscles and acupuncture points, which is consistent with clinical guideline recommendations (see Chapter 2). It is important to note that, when performing *tuina* 推拿 therapy, strong stimulation should be avoided to prevent potential injury of the joint capsule.

Cupping therapy has been proved effective when used as an add-on therapy for shoulder pain. Mobile cupping on the painful area

Table 10.4 Summary of Other Chinese Medicine Therapies

Other Chinese Medicine Therapy Type	Included in Clinical Guidelines and Textbooks (Chapter 2)	Included in Classical Literature (Chapter 3) (No. of Citations)	Evidence in Clinical Studies (Chapter 8) (No. of Studies)			Included in Combination Therapies (Chapter 9) (No. of Studies)
			RCTs	CCTs	Non-controlled Studies	
Tuina 推拿 therapy	Yes	0	9	0	4	14
Cupping therapy	No	0	2	0	0	1

Abbreviations: CCTs, controlled clinical trials; RCTs, randomised controlled trials.

during shoulder movement could reduce pain symptoms and improve upper limb function.

Practitioners wishing to use these therapies for post-stroke shoulder complications should consider this in light of the available evidence.

Limitations of the Evidence

Although considerable effort was made to identify data from a wide range of sources, there may have been limitations from each of the data resources.

In Chapter 2, since we did not identify any CM clinical guideline or textbook introducing post-stroke shoulder complications as an independent condition, the CM treatments specifically targeting post-stroke shoulder complications are lacking. Therefore, we combined clinical experts' opinions and the recommendations from a number of clinical guidelines and textbooks. The main feature of treatments listed in Chapter 2, particularly CHM treatments, is that they were focused on post-stroke motor function impairment and pain. It is possible that readers may consider some other treatments are also effective for these complications.

The analyses of the classical literature (Chapter 3) were based on a large sample of CM books which are included in *Zhong Hua Yi Dian* 中华医典 version 5. Our assessment indicates that this was the largest available digital resource available at the time, but it does not include every CM book published in pre-modern eras so omissions are inevitable. The search processes employed a number of different search terms, but we could not be certain that all relevant citations were located and included in the analyses. Since the citations were written by multiple individuals over the course of history, there have been changes in language usage and meaning, and errors have crept into the processes involved in copying and printing manuscripts. Therefore, it is likely that the intended meaning of some citations has been misinterpreted and/or mistranslated. Similarly, the identity of some herbs can change over time and with geographical position so it is possible that regularisation errors have been made in the allocation of scientific names. Moreover, considering there has not been any disease name referring to post-stroke shoulder complications, the analyses of CM treatment in classical literature are based on symptoms of post-stroke motor function impairment with the presence of upper limb symptoms. Therefore, the results of classical literature analyses may not be consistent with what are in use currently. Also, it is not accurate to assume that the most frequently used herbs represent the most effective treatments because there is no method to evaluate the efficacy. What they represent is a short list of herbs that could be considered for further research.

The clinical trial evidence was based on searches of multiple databases and resulted in thousands of search results. Since there was considerable variation in the conditions under which these trials were conducted, the age and severity of the participants, the frequency and duration of interventions, and the procedures used in data collection and analysis, it was not surprising that statistical heterogeneity tended to be 'high', although random effects models were used. Where possible, subgroup analyses were conducted but they did not reduce the heterogeneity. The quality of the reporting of the methodological details of trial design and conduct was not adequate in many studies. Most of the included studies did not report proper random sequence generation. Blinding had not been applied and there was inadequate information on drop outs and adverse events in the majority of studies.

For each category of evidence, frequency tables are provided that summarise the most commonly used interventions, including the herbal formula names, the herbal ingredients used in the formulas and the acupuncture points used in the clinical studies. Due to the large volume of available data, presentation of the details of every study was not feasible and these tables only included the interventions that were the most frequently used. Lower frequency interventions may not be mentioned unless they feature prominently in the meta-analyses. Also, it should not be inferred that the most frequently used interventions were the most effective ones.

The majority of included clinical studies compared the combination of CM therapy and routine care/rehabilitation to routine care/rehabilitation alone. In such studies, there was often a benefit for the combination therapy, particularly when no placebo for the CM therapy was used and the study was not blinded. Due to the lack of blinding, the efficacy results achieved may not reflect the real therapeutic effects of CM therapies, since there is the possibly that there have been non-specific effects caused by adding an additional treatment.

The above limitations should be taken in consideration when interpreting the data included in the previous chapters.

Implications for Practice

In the traditional manner, CM practice is inherited from the records in previous literature or senior practitioners' clinical experience. The evidence-based practice approach was not adopted for the development of textbooks or clinical practice guidelines in CM. In this research, we evaluated evidence from classical literature and current clinical research, and provided information on how, and to what extent, treatments of post-stroke shoulder complications were developed. The research provides evidence which supports the recommendation for the use of CM therapies, and identified the gap between contemporary literature and current clinical practice, in terms of some treatment methods.

Historically, post-stroke shoulder complications were not addressed as independent clinical conditions. Therefore, relevant treatments were identified from citations of stroke (*zhong feng* 中风). The word *zhong feng* 中风 refers to 'a sudden Wind attack'. The concept of 'Wind' in stroke was initially an external pathogen which then developed to be internal factors. In particular, the treatment purposes of tonifying *qi* 气, removing Blood stasis and opening up meridians are consistent with that of *Bu yang huan wu tang* 补阳还五汤, a formula introduced by a book published in the Qing dynasty. This is also the key formula being recommended by clinical guidelines to treat post-stroke functional impairment. The clinical trial evidence, in particular the evidence from RCTs, provides the best available evidence for the effectiveness of particular CM interventions. Although there was insufficient evidence to support the effects of reducing the acromiohumeral interval in shoulder subluxation, adding CM therapies to routine care/rehabilitation is generally beneficial for relieving pain, improving upper limb function or patients' daily activities.

Findings from reviews of clinical evidence suggest that CHM, acupuncture therapies, *tuina* 推拿 and cupping therapies could be incorporated into an overall health care plan for post-stroke shoulder complications, in particular being used as add-on therapies to routine care and rehabilitation. The quality of evidence was assessed for the main therapies using the GRADE approach. With caution regarding the limitation of the evidence stated above, it was concluded that:

- Topical CHM appeared to be an effective add-on therapy for shoulder pain (GRADE: 'very low' to 'low') and SHS (GRADE: 'very low' to 'low');
- Acupuncture appeared to be an effective add-on therapy for shoulder subluxation (GRADE: 'very low' to 'low'), shoulder pain (GRADE: 'low' to 'moderate'), and SHS (GRADE: 'low');
- Electroacupuncture appeared to be an effective add-on therapy for shoulder subluxation (GRADE: 'low') and SHS (GRADE: 'low' to 'moderate').

CHM formulas in clinical studies were selected, or modified, with a focus on pain relief, which reflects the main symptom of post-stroke shoulder complications. There is more clinical evidence supporting the use of topical CHM than oral CHM. CHM was often administered in the forms of CHM bath therapy, CHM fomentation, CHM steam therapy and CHM external application.

Acupuncture and moxibustion therapies have been consistently recorded in all forms of literature, with the point LI15 *Jianyu* 肩髃

being the most promising one. Clinical evidence also showed the benefit of some modern-style acupuncture therapies, although they were not mentioned in classical literature or clinical guidelines. Clinicians should use their clinical judgment when considering these techniques for people with post-stroke shoulder complications. *Tuina* 推拿 therapy seems to play an important role in the management of post-stroke shoulder complications.

Implications for Research

CM therapies are increasingly evaluated through clinical trials, in line with the development of Western medicine. Our systematic analyses found that the CM managements of post-stroke shoulder complications are consistent and encouraging, but 'high' quality evidence is lacking. Hence, there is a need for well-designed clinical trials of CM interventions in order to provide reliable assessment of treatment effects. Further high-quality clinical trials are needed which address the following priority aspects:

General Trial Design

- Randomised controlled trials should be designed with rigorous methodology, with particular attention paid to adequate randomisation and allocation concealment;
- Since CM therapies are commonly administered as add-on therapies to routine care/rehabilitation, efforts should be made to ensure blinding of participants and practitioners with the use of placebo or sham controls;
- Clinical trial protocols should be registered in Clinical Trial Registries, or be published prior to the conduct of RCTs, to increase transparency in reporting;
- Considering post-stroke shoulder complications are a long-term condition, long-term effects of CM therapies for post-stroke shoulder complications should be evaluated in a follow-up phase using well-validated outcome measures.

Intervention and Control

- For CHM, authentication of raw material should be described, and for manufactured products, reports should include the quantity of active constituents;
- Syndrome differentiation should be considered in study design to improve applicability in clinical practice;
- Placebo controls for CHM should be applied in testing the add-on effects of integrating CHM with routine care. While for acupuncture and other manual therapies, the difficulties in blinding the person delivering the therapy are well known, it is still feasible to blind the participants using a sham device.[1,2]

Reporting

- Research reports should follow the CONSORT statement with reference to the extension for herbal medicine[3] and STRICTA for clinical trials of acupuncture;[4]
- Individual modifications of the CHM formula or acupuncture points should be reported with more detail, in order to instruct real-life clinical practice;
- Any modification, or adjustment, to the treatment method recommended by current clinical guidelines, and why and how these are done, should be addressed when reporting the results.

Diversity was seen in the range of CM therapies, both within and across forms of evidence, reflecting the nature of CM clinical practice. Future research should focus on the most promising findings identified, and investigate the efficacy and safety of those therapies that are feasible to be widely used in clinical practice.

The consistency with which certain herbs were used as ingredients in classical formulas (Chapter 3) and in clinical trials (Chapters 5 and 9) was highlighted by the herb frequency analyses in each of these chapters. As Chapter 6 briefly summarised, there has been a number of experimental studies on the frequently used herbs which have demonstrated bio-activities that are relevant to post-stroke shoulder complications and may, at least, partially explain how the herbal formulas could have acted. Future studies could assess the effects of these herbs, and their constituent compounds in various combinations, as they are commonly used in the formulas.

References

1. Zhang CS, Yang AW, Zhang AL, *et al.* (2014) Sham control methods used in ear-acupuncture/ear-acupressure randomized controlled trials: A systematic review. *J Altern Complem Med* **20**(3): 147–161.
2. Zhang CS, Tan HY, Zhang GS, *et al.* (2015) Placebo devices as effective control methods in acupuncture clinical trials: A systematic review. *PLoS One* **10**(11): e0140825.
3. Pandis N, Chung B, Scherer RW, *et al.* (2017) CONSORT 2010 statement: Extension checklist for reporting within person randomised trials. *BMJ* **357**: j2835.
4. MacPherson H, White A, Cummings M, *et al.* (2001) Standards for reporting interventions in controlled trials of acupuncture: The STRICTA recommendations. *Complement Ther Med* **9**(4): 246–249.

Glossary

Glossary of Terms	Acronym	Definition	Reference
95% confidence interval	95% CI	A measure of the uncertainty around the main finding of a statistical analysis. Estimates of unknown quantities, such as the odds ratio comparing an experimental intervention with a control, are usually presented as a point estimate and a 95% confidence interval. This means that if someone were to keep repeating a study in other samples from the same population, 95% of the confidence intervals from those studies would contain the true value of the unknown quantity. Alternatives to 95%, such as 90% and 99% confidence intervals, are sometimes used. Wider intervals indicate lower precision; narrow intervals, greater precision.	http://handbook.cochrane.org/
Acupressure	—	Application of pressure to acupuncture points.	—
Acupuncture	—	The insertion of needles into humans or animals for remedial purposes or its methods.	World Health Organisation. (2007) WHO International Standard Terminologies of Traditional Medicine in the Western Pacific Region.
Acromiohumeral Interval	AHI	The shortest distance measured between the inferior cortex (dense line) of the acromion and the humerus.	—

(Continued)

(Continued)

Glossary of Terms	Acronym	Definition	Reference
Allied and Complementary Medicine Database	AMED	Alternative medicine bibliographic database.	https://www.ebscohost.com/academic/AMED-The-Allied-and-Complementary-Medicine-Database
Barthel Index	BI	A simple tool for assessing self-care and mobility, consisting of ten common activities of daily living, administered through direct observation.	—
China National Knowledge Infrastructure	CNKI	Chinese language bibliographic database.	www.cnki.net
Chinese Biomedical Literature Database	CBM	Chinese language bibliographic database.	https://cbmwww.imicams.ac.cn
Chinese herbal medicine	CHM	—	—
Chinese medicine	CM	—	—
Chongqing VIP Information Company	CQVIP	Chinese language bibliographic database.	www.cqvip
ClinicalTrials.gov	—	Clinical Trial Registry.	https://clinicaltrials.gov/
Cochrane Central Register of Controlled Trials	CENTRAL	Bibliographic database that provides a highly concentrated source of reports of randomised controlled trials.	http://community.cochrane.org/editorial-and-publishing-policy-resource/cochrane-central-register-controlled-trials-central
Combination therapies	—	Two or more Chinese medicines from different therapy groups (CHM, acupuncture therapies or other CM therapies) administered together.	—
Convention on International Trade in Endangered Species of Wild Fauna and Flora	CITES	—	https://www.cites.org/eng/disc/text.php
Cumulative Index of Nursing and Allied Health Literature	CINAHL	Bibliographic database.	https://www.ebscohost.com/nursing/about

(Continued)

(*Continued*)

Glossary of Terms	Acronym	Definition	Reference
Cupping therapy	—	Suction by using a vacuumised cup or jar.	World Health Organisation. (2007) WHO International Standard Terminologies of Traditional Medicine in the Western Pacific Region.
Effect size	—	A generic term for the estimate of effect of treatment for a study.	http://handbook.cochrane.org/
Effective rate	ER	A measure of the proportion of participants who achieved an improvement, as outlined in the Methods for evaluating clinical evidence section.	—
Electroacupuncture	—	Electric stimulation of the needle following insertion.	World Health Organisation. (2007) WHO International Standard Terminologies of Traditional Medicine in the Western Pacific Region.
Excerpta Medica dataBASE	Embase	Bibliographic database.	http://www.elsevier.com/solutions/embase
Fugl-Meyer Assessment	FMA	A disease-specific impairment index designed to assess motor function, balance, sensation qualities and joint function in hemiplegic post-stroke patients.	—
Grading of Recommendations Assessment, Development and Evaluation	GRADE	Approach to grading quality of evidence and strength of recommendations.	http://www.gradeworkinggroup.org/
Heterogeneity	—	1. Used in a general sense to describe the variation in, or diversity of, participants, interventions and measurement of outcomes across a set of studies, or the variation in internal validity of those studies. 2. Used specifically, as statistical heterogeneity, to describe the degree of variation in the	http://handbook.cochrane.org/

(*Continued*)

(*Continued*)

Glossary of Terms	Acronym	Definition	Reference
		effect estimates from a set of studies. Also used to indicate the presence of variability among studies beyond the amount expected due solely to the play of chance.	
I^2	—	A measure of study heterogeneity; indicates the percentage of variance in a meta-analysis.	http://handbook.cochrane.org/
Integrative medicine	—	The combined use of a Chinese medicine treatment with conventional medical management.	—
Mean difference	MD	In meta-analysis, a method used to combine measures on continuous scales, where the mean, standard deviation and sample size in each group are known. The weight given to the difference in means from each study (e.g. how much influence each study has on the overall results of the meta-analysis) is determined by the precision of its estimate of effect; mathematically this is equal to the inverse of the variance. This method assumes that all of the trials have measured the outcome on the same scale.	http://handbook.cochrane.org/
Meta-analysis	—	The use of statistical techniques in a systematic review to integrate the results of included studies. Sometimes misused as a synonym for systematic reviews, where the review includes a meta-analysis.	—

(*Continued*)

(*Continued*)

Glossary of Terms	Acronym	Definition	Reference
Moxibustion	—	A therapeutic procedure involving ignited material (usually moxa) to apply heat to certain points or areas of the body surface for curing disease through regulation of the function of meridians/channels and visceral organs.	World Health Organisation. (2007) WHO International Standard Terminologies of Traditional Medicine in the Western Pacific Region.
Non-controlled studies	—	Observations made on individuals, usually receiving the same intervention, before and after an intervention but with no control group.	http://handbook.cochrane.org/
Non-randomised controlled clinical trials	CCT	An experimental study in which people are allocated to different interventions using methods that are not random.	http://handbook.cochrane.org/
Other Chinese medicine therapies	—	Other Chinese medicine therapies include all traditional therapies except Chinese herbal medicine and acupuncture, e.g. tai chi, qigong, Chinese pulmonary rehabilitation, *tuina* 推拿 and cupping.	—
PubMed	PubMed	Bibliographic database.	http://www.ncbi.nlm.nih.gov/pubmed
Randomised controlled trial	RCT	—	—
Range of motion	ROM	—	—
Risk of bias	—	Assessment of clinical trials to indicate if the results may overestimate or underestimate the true effect because of bias in study design or reporting.	http://handbook.cochrane.org/
Risk ratio	RR	The ratio of risks in two groups. In intervention studies, it is the ratio of the risk in the intervention group to the risk in the control group. A risk ratio of 1 indicates no difference between	http://handbook.cochrane.org/

(*Continued*)

249

(Continued)

Glossary of Terms	Acronym	Definition	Reference
		comparison groups. For undesirable outcomes, a risk ratio that is less than 1 indicates that the intervention was effective in reducing the risk of that outcome.	
Standardised mean difference	SMD	In meta-analysis, a method used to combine results for continuous scales which measure the same outcome, but in different ways (e.g. with different scales). The results of studies are standardised to a uniform scale to allow data to be combined.	http://handbook.cochrane.org/
Summary of findings	SoF	Presentation of results and rating the quality of evidence based on the GRADE approach.	http://www.gradeworkinggroup.org/
Tuina 推拿	—	Chinese massage: rubbing, kneading or percussion of the soft tissues and joints of the body with the hands, usually performed by one person on another, especially to relieve tension or pain.	World Health Organisation. (2007) WHO International Standard Terminologies of Traditional Medicine in the Western Pacific Region.
Visual Analogue Scale	VAS	A commonly used unidimensional measurement instrument to measure pain intensity.	—
Wanfang database	Wanfang	Chinese language bibliographic database.	www.wanfangdata.com
World Health Organisation	WHO	WHO is the directing and coordinating authority for health within the United Nations system. It is responsible for providing leadership on global health matters, shaping the health research agenda, setting	http://www.who.int/about/en/

(Continued)

Glossary

Glossary of Terms	Acronym	Definition	Reference
		norms and standards, articulating evidence-based policy options, providing technical support to countries and monitoring and assessing health trends.	
Zhong Hua Yi Dian	ZHYD	The Zhong Hua Yi Dian (ZHYD) (Encyclopaedia of Traditional Chinese Medicine) is a comprehensive series of electronic books on compact disk. The collection was put together by the Hunan electronic and audio-visual publishing house. It is the largest collection of Chinese electronic books and includes the major Chinese classical works, many of which are from rare manuscripts and are the only existing copies. These books cover the period from before the Tang dynasty to the period of the Republic of China (1911–1948).	Hu R, ed. (2000) Zhong Hua Yi Dian [Encyclopaedia of Traditional Chinese Medicine], 4th ed. Hunan Electronic and Audio-Visual Publishing House, Chengsha.

Index

Evidence-based Clinical Chinese Medicine

Print ISSN: 2529-7562
Online ISSN: 2529-7554

Series Co Editors-in-Chief

Charlie Changli Xue *(RMIT University, Australia)*
Chuanjian Lu *(Guangdong Provincial Hospital of Chinese Medicine, China)*

Published

More information on this series can also be found at https://www.worldscientific.com/series/ebccm